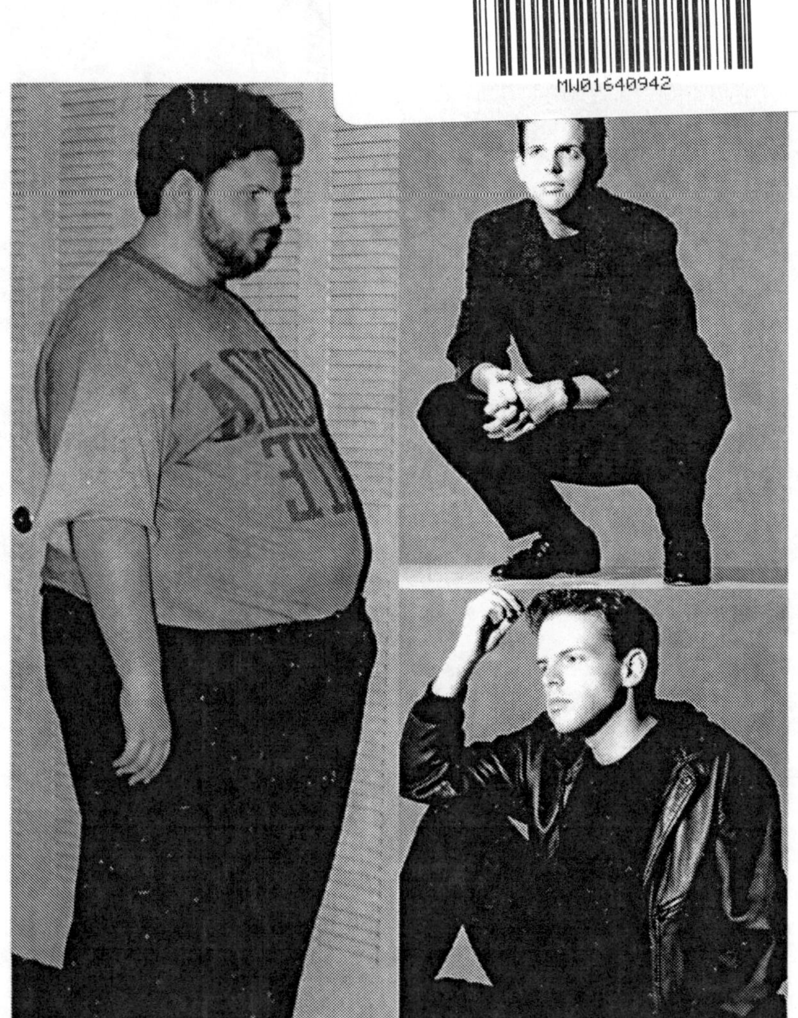

Just Stop Eating So Much!

The No-Excuses Way to Lose Weight and Feel Great

By Gregg McBride

NOTICE:
Just Stop Eating So Much! is intended as a reference only, not as a medical manual. The information given here is designed to help you make informed decisions about your health. It is not intended as a substitute for any treatment that may have been prescribed by your doctor. If you suspect you have a medical condition, you are urged to seek competent medical help.

Also, mention of specific companies, organizations or authorities does not imply endorsement by Just Stop Eating So Much!, nor does mention of specific companies, organizations or authorities imply that they endorse Just Stop Eating So Much!

Internet addresses and other references listed in Just Stop Eating So Much! were accurate at the time it went to press.

Just Stop Eating So Much!

ISBN: 978-0-6151-4831-1

Dedicated to everyone
who's ever tried to change
his or her life.

This time you're really
going to do it.

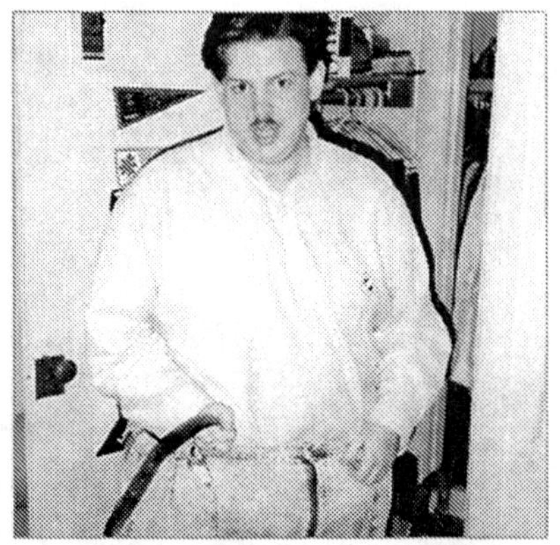

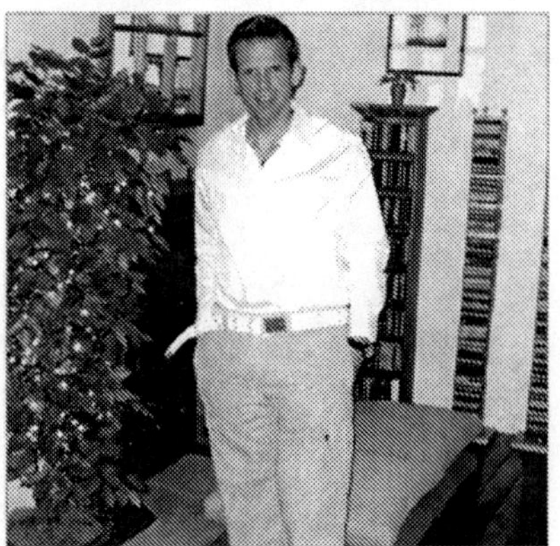

Contents

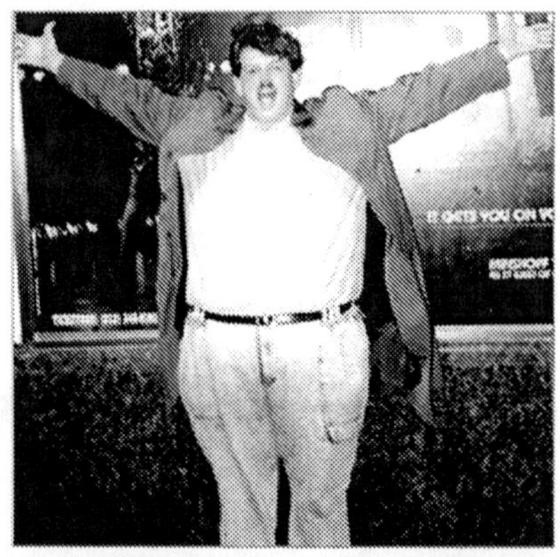

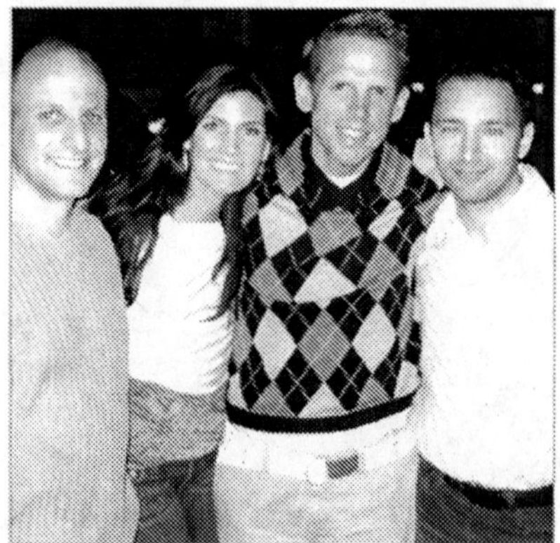

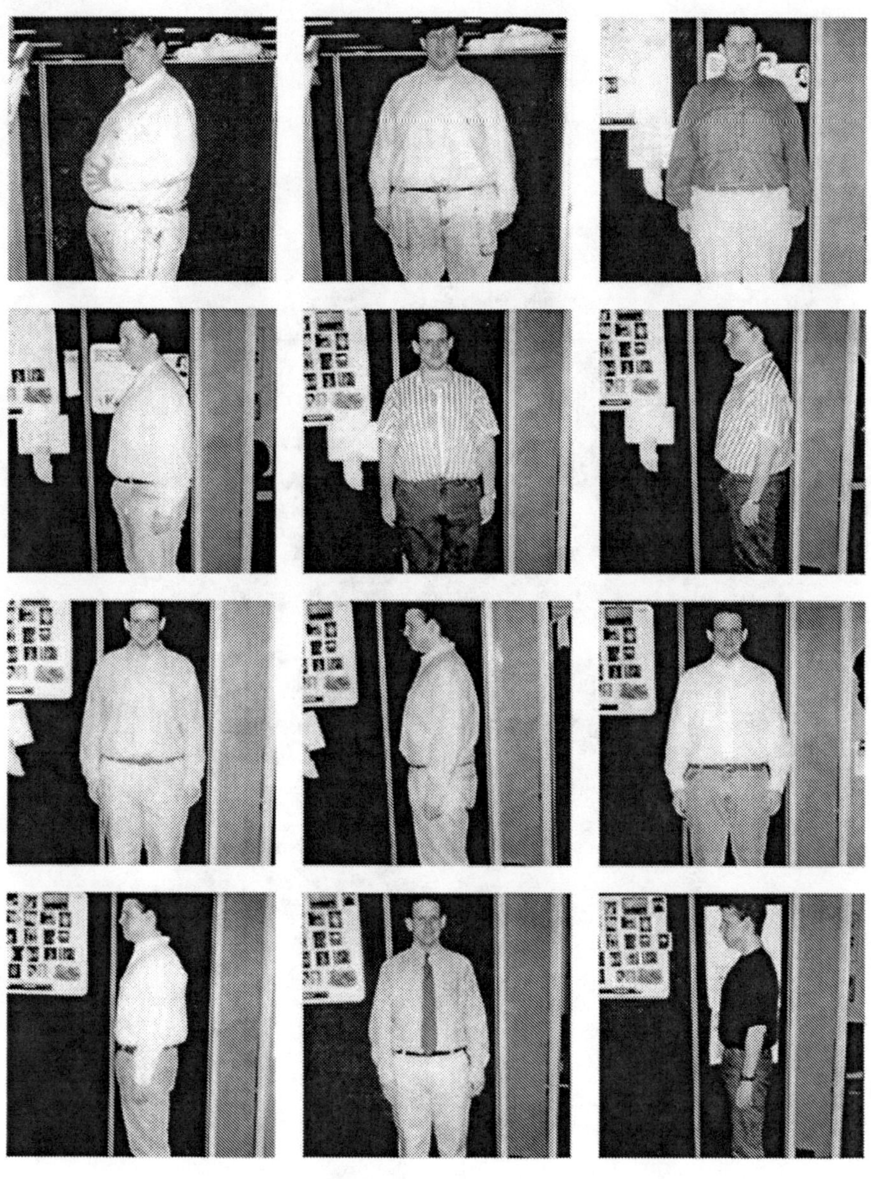

Starting Weight: 450+ lbs
(*the scale wouldn't go any higher*)

Ending Weight: 175 lbs

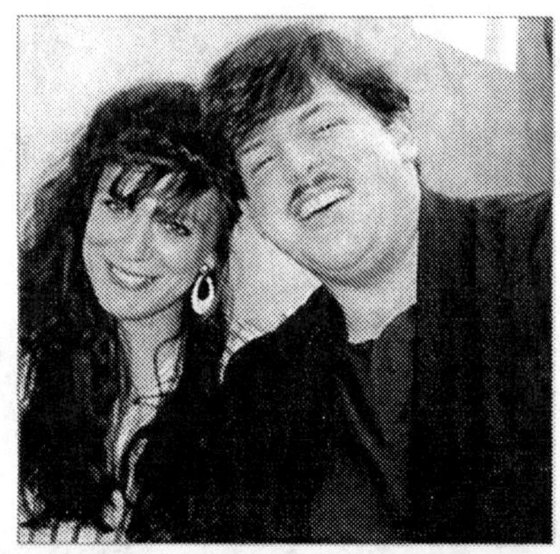

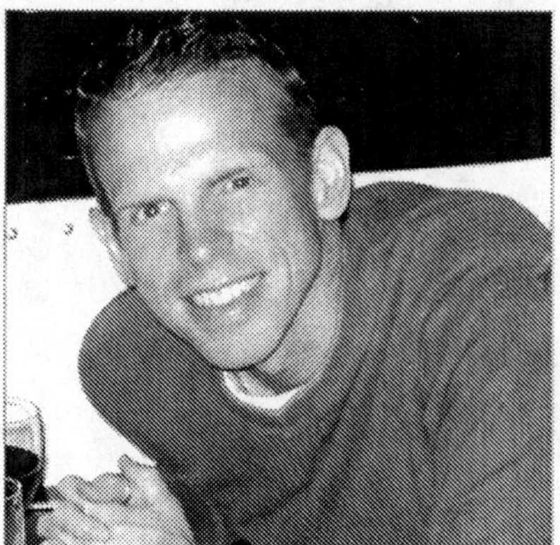

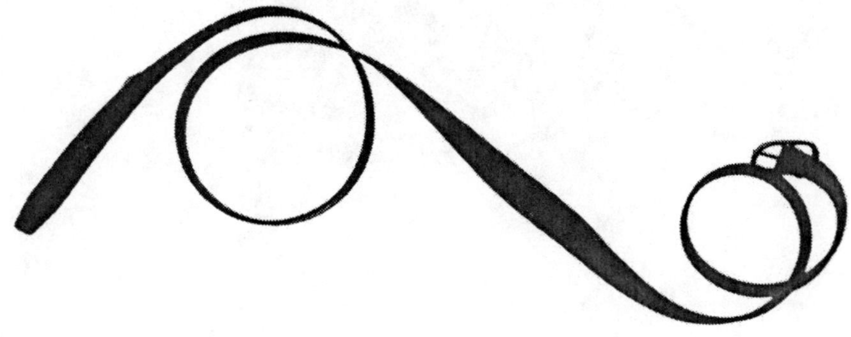

Meet My Belt…

The belt you see here is for a 60-inch waist. If you ever meet me in person, ask to see it. I'll show you how it was worn down around the belt buckle holes – from when it was keeping my 60-plus-inch waist from spilling out over my pants, or popping buttons on my shirt. Even though I haven't needed this belt for well over 10 years, I keep it as a reminder of what I accomplished – and I share it as a promise of what *you* can accomplish.

And the best news? You won't need surgery…or pills…or the latest fad…or a personal trainer…or a private chef…or an expensive food delivery service. You have *everything* you need right here!

Before I took control and created the Just Stop Eating So Much! Plan, I had been overweight for most of my life. I have memories of eating too much and stuffing my face from as far back as the first grade. My parents were horrified and tried to put me on all kinds of diets (even at age six!), and they banned candy and snacks from the house.

Well, I showed them! Eating "forbidden food" became my way to rebel. And rebel I did.

By the time I was a senior in high school, I had ballooned to an enormous weight and had been known as "the fat, funny kid" for most of my life. (Note which descriptor came first!)

Here's my high school senior class picture. I was trying to look sexy. Looking back, I think I look a little sad:

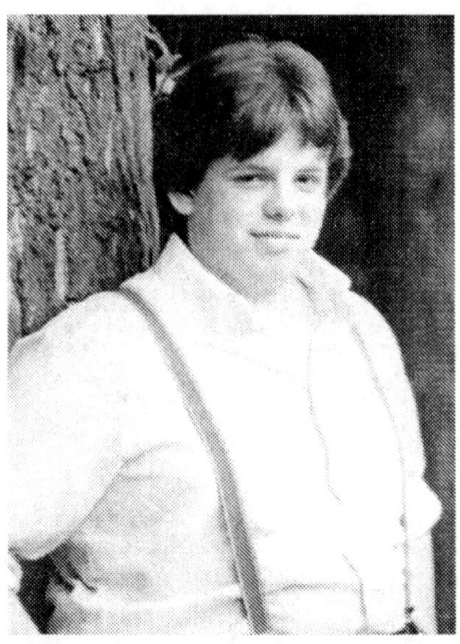

Even though people thought of me as the class clown (a title I wore proudly – anything to gain some much desired popularity), inside I yearned to be as good looking as some of the jocks and cheerleaders I had become friends with. I knew I was heavy, but tried my hardest to look as good as possible. I used to get dressed for school and ask my sister, "Am I F-F-A-F-K?" This translated to, "Am I Foxy For a Fat Kid?" I'm not sure *where* I got that terminology. Maybe from watching one too many rerun of some 1970s sitcom. But you get the idea.

I was desperate to fit in (no pun intended). And I was trying to lose weight. I would put myself on various types of diets and even temporary fasts.

I remember one time going a whole week on diet and starting to feel better about myself, and then finding a half-eaten bag of potato chips in the kitchen trash can. If you're wondering if I ate them, the answer is… "Yes." That's right – I ate junk food out of the trash. The diets weren't working. And I decided the reason for that was that there was something wrong with me.

Sadly, high school wasn't the end of my "growing" phase.

By the time I graduated from college, despite a lifetime of dieting attempts (usually I'd lose several pounds, then gain back even more weight), I found myself weighing more than 450 pounds. Eating was pretty much my sole focus in life. Even though I knew it was killing me – literally. I was living a life in Purgatory.

And yet I couldn't find any solution for my problem. No matter how many diet books I read, no matter how many weight loss groups or organizations I joined, no matter how much money I spent, I just kept getting fatter.

Here I am right after college graduation...still smiling (and with a perm – yikes!). I actually remember being out of breath while this picture was taken – even though I was just standing there:

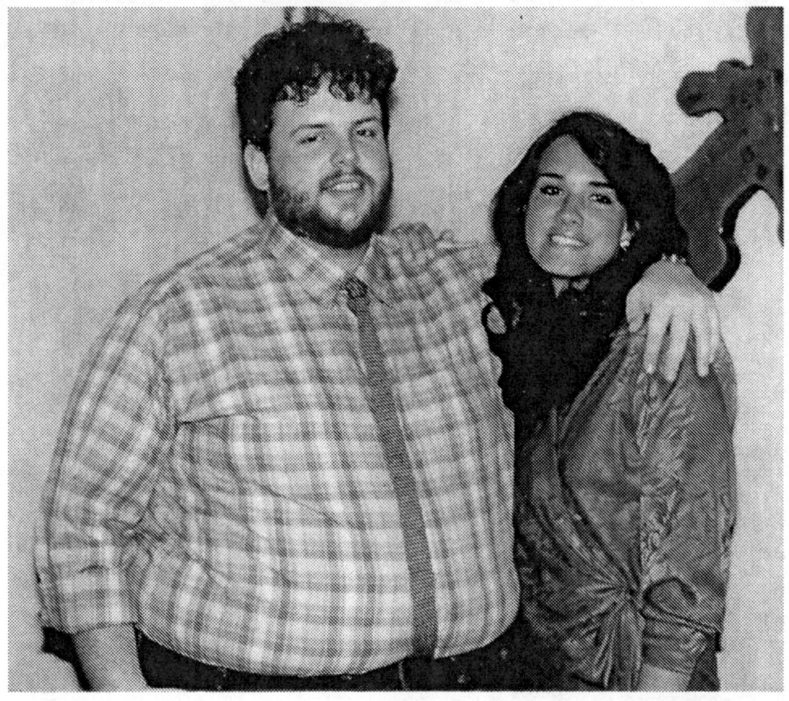

I want to emphasize that I'm not saying "Poor me." I realize *I* was the one putting the food in my mouth. But the fact is that our society *does* treat fat people with a lot of resentment, hatred and misunderstanding. You might even know what I'm talking about… People treated me like I had a disease and wouldn't even look me in the eye.

I remember going on job interviews (after just graduating from college) and having prospective employers not hire me because they assumed I was lazy and unmotivated. How could they know that? Was it just because of my size?

I also know the misery of weighing so much that just talking on the phone would leave me breathless – as well as the misery of having no social life and no chance of any kind of romantic relationship. I remember being forced to shop for ugly clothes and often not being able to find anything that fit comfortably – even in the "big and tall" stores.

I remember boarding an airplane and having to ask for an extension for my seatbelt (as well as witness the horror of the person who realized he or she was going to have to sit next to someone so heavy during a cross-country flight). I remember the food binges, too – those times I was by myself, eating as much as I could as a way to stop the pain of being a fat man in a thin society. Fact is, I hated myself more than anyone else did.

Here I am celebrating Christmas in New York…shortly before turning my back on the diet industry and deciding to take the weight off *myself*:

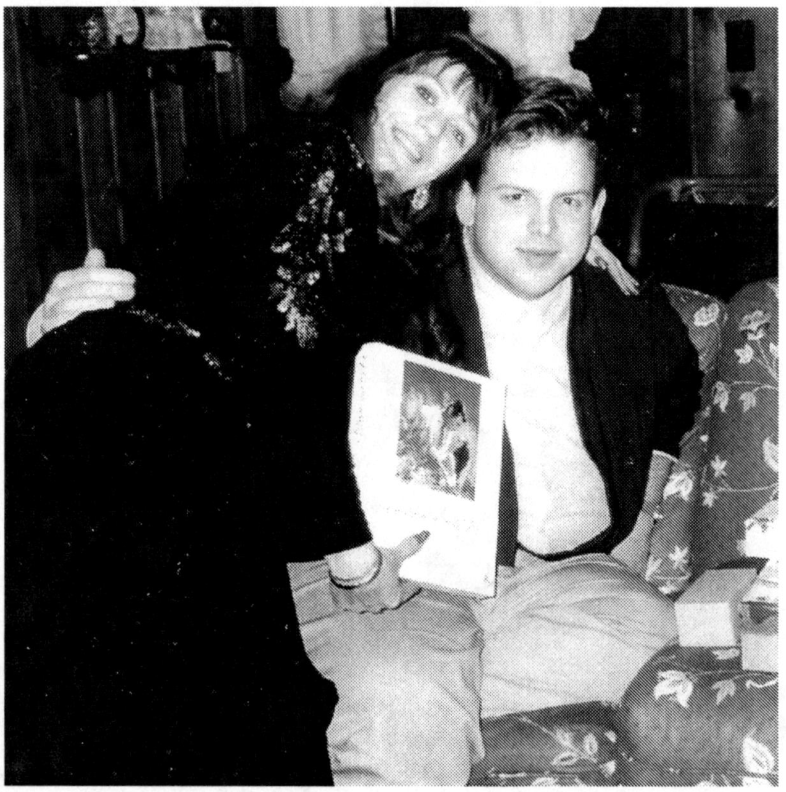

Anyone who has weight to lose knows how much willpower it takes to try (and try again!) every diet known to man – including some very dangerous diets – in an effort to just fit in with the rest of society.

Like many of you, I tried all the different diets out there. I was determined to be the poster boy for some weight loss group or organization. But it seemed the more I tried, the fatter I got.

Sure, I'd lose a couple pounds initially. But then I'd gain even more weight back. And when I asked about it, the so called authorities of these weight loss groups or organizations would encourage me to start again or rejoin. *Restart the diet plan on which I just gained 10 pounds?* But yeah, I did rejoin…and usually gained more on top of that (after the initial loss).

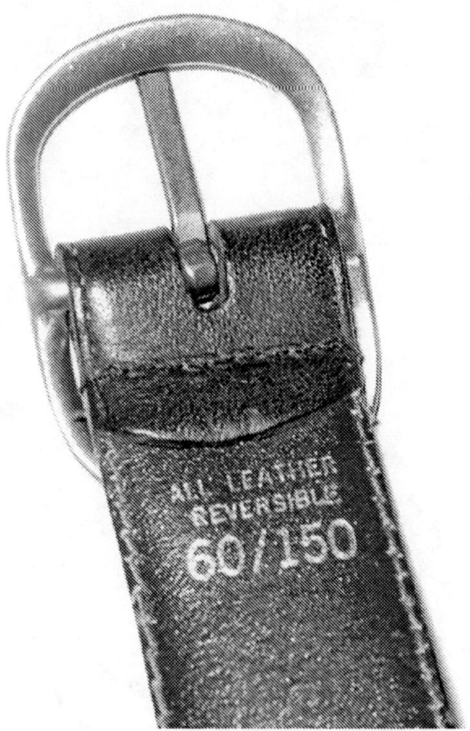

It wasn't until I took matters into my own hands that I made a life change that resulted in my taking off more than 250 pounds in less than a year's time – and then keeping it off for more than ten years, up until this day. People who meet me now tell me they never could imagine I weighed as much as I did. Or that I wore a belt that was for a 60" waist. But I did. And I share this belt with you as a symbol of what you can achieve – no matter how much excess weight you want to take off.

You can forget the baloney that the diet industry has been selling you. You can achieve your goals without surgery, without pills, without fads, without a personal trainer, without a personal chef and without special food delivery services. Together with Just Stop Eating So Much! you can do it *yourself*!

I can't wait for you to share the picture of your "Before Belt" with me. In fact, I'll want to hear all of your stories and about your success. You're holding something in your hands that will change your life if you let it. It all starts with a commitment – to yourself.

I believe in *you*.

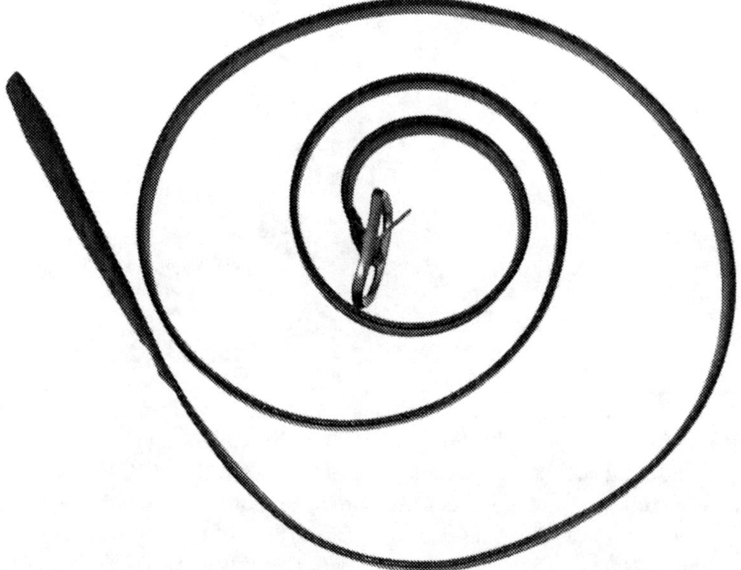

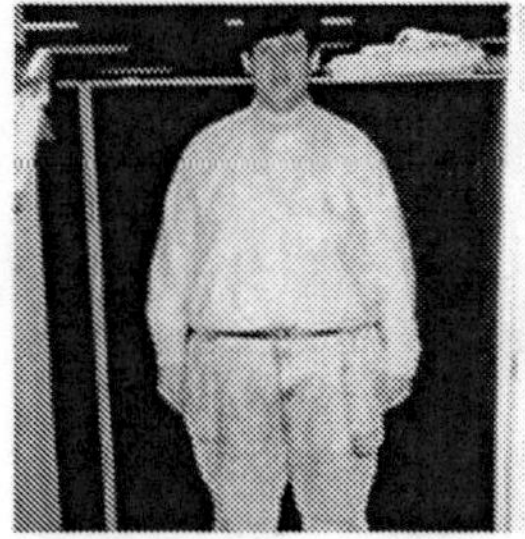

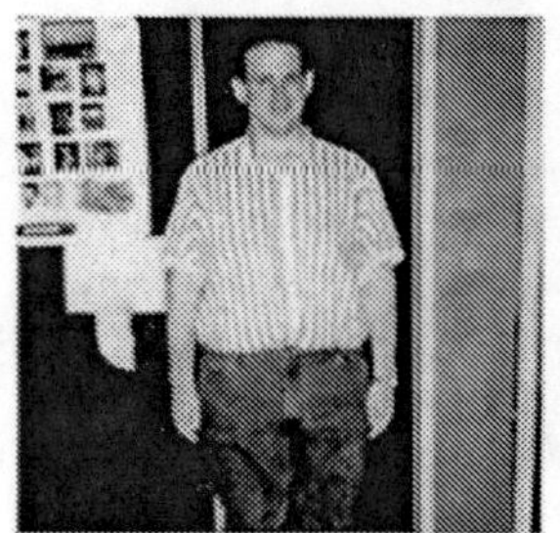

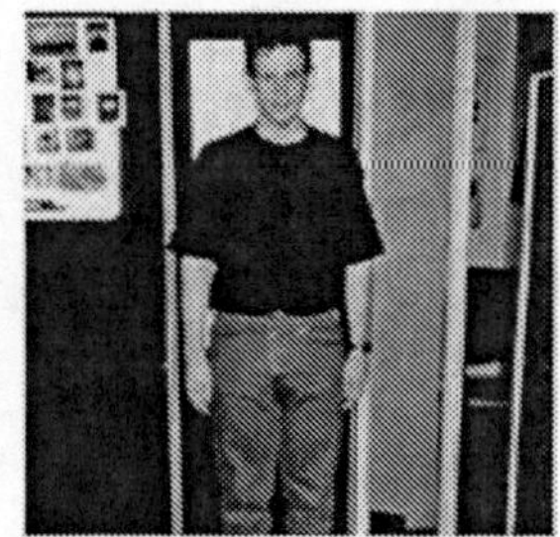

Introduction

For ages, men and women have pondered the mystery of how to lose their excess weight. They've joined weight loss groups, paid for expensive nutritionists, hired personal chefs, enlisted over-caffeinated trainers, forked over tons of cash for expensive meal delivery services, altered their bodies with dangerous surgeries, taken pills and even starved themselves – all in an effort to get thinner, look better and feel healthier.

I can't seem to stop eating.

I think my metabolism is too slow.

I can't eat carbs.

I need a quick fix.

I'll be able to lose weight after the holidays.

I'll never be able to fit into a smaller clothing size.

I don't have any willpower.

I can't do it myself.

As a winner of the *weight*-ing game, I'm here to say that despite your good intentions to be thinner and healthier, you've been wasting your time. Losing weight isn't complicated, although the $4 billion a year diet industry would like you think it is.

The ways to feeling and looking better are simple. And you've known them all along.

The *secret* to losing weight and looking great? **Just Stop Eating So Much!**

Unfortunately, people have become so brainwashed by society, they now look for quick fixes and "tricks" to take off the pounds. It's not about being sensible anymore. The media, diet centers, nutritionists and even doctors and surgeons have us convinced that losing weight is a mystery…A mystery that's going to cost your life savings – and, quite possibly, your *life* – to solve.

After a lifetime of trying fad diets, joining hundreds of diet programs, seeing doctors, considering surgeries, fasting, eliminating carbs, combining certain food groups, and depriving and hurting my body in an attempt to shed what became over 250 pounds of excess weight, I finally realized something amazing: The more I tried to find the "magic pill" for losing weight, the more pounds I packed on. When I graduated from college, I literally tipped the scales at 450 pounds (that's as high as my scale went – above that weight my electronic scale read "Error" – or, as I like to put it, "Get off!").

That's when **Just Stop Eating So Much!** became my rule of thumb (and *mouth*). By embracing simple truths of eating, moving (it's called "exercise," people) and working on my self-esteem, I got back to the basics and the weight began to melt off. Within a year, I had "released" more than 250 pounds. (I never call it "losing" weight because I never want it back!)

While friends and even strangers witnessed my miraculous change, they all asked me for the *secret*.

What magic pill was I taking?

What weight loss group did I belong to?

What diet guru was I seeing?

What Hollywood trainer was working with me?

What kind of surgery did I have performed?

What pact had I made with the devil?

No one (*no one!*) believed me when I revealed my mysterious solution... I was eating less and exercising more.

No, it wasn't easy – but nothing in life is. And I was no longer risking my life on fad diets, sitting in a room full of people confessing why I had cheated on my "Eating Plan," eliminating certain food groups my body needs to function, taking pills, starving myself…or having metal objects inserted into my gut to keep my stomach from being able to hold more than a hard-boiled egg.

I *just stopped eating so much*! And took off more than 250 pounds – and have kept the excess weight off for over 10 years.

I'm the first to admit that this "simple" strategy was, indeed, one of the most difficult to grasp. That's why after years of having people literally beg me to share my method, my story, my motivation, my *success*, and after years of helping my friends achieve their weight loss goals, I'm putting all of my *simple secrets* in one easy-to-follow book. After all, I've kept the weight off for years and have never looked better. My skin glows, my eyes shine and my health is perfect. The sun shines brighter whenever I'm around. (Okay… Not really. But you get the idea!) That's because I gave up the dieting tricks and went for the real thing: *common sense*.

Just Stop Eating So Much! is a provocative, hilarious, and, above all, intoxicatingly liberating approach to taking off the excess pounds and getting your life back. It deserves a place in everyone's life.

I know you're an amazing, powerful, beautiful, healthy, *thin* person who has everything it takes inside to look great on the outside. No surgery, pills or medically risky ways of life required!

The next time you start wondering what's wrong with you, and why, after all these years and all that money, you can't seem to take the weight off, reach for this book – it holds the simple answers, the simple food plans, the simple exercise regimes, the simple self-esteem builders…The simple *truths*.

Just Stop Eating So Much! is here to change your life… *Forever*!

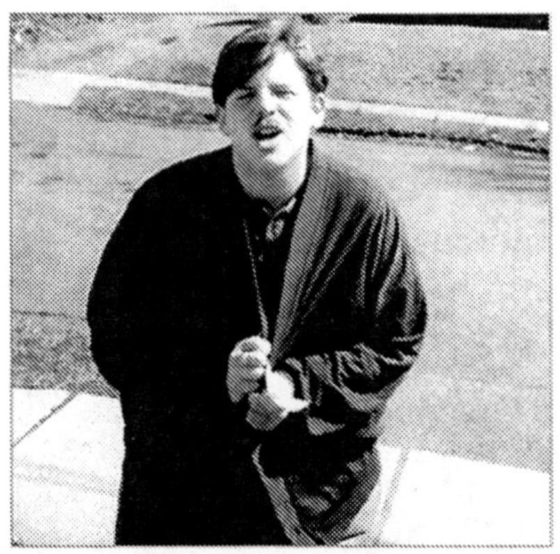

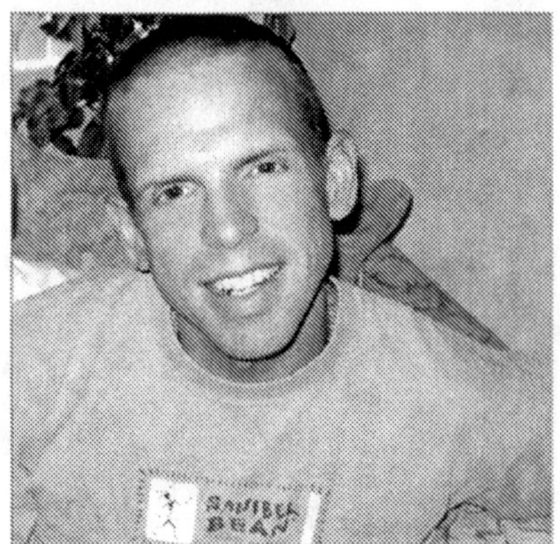

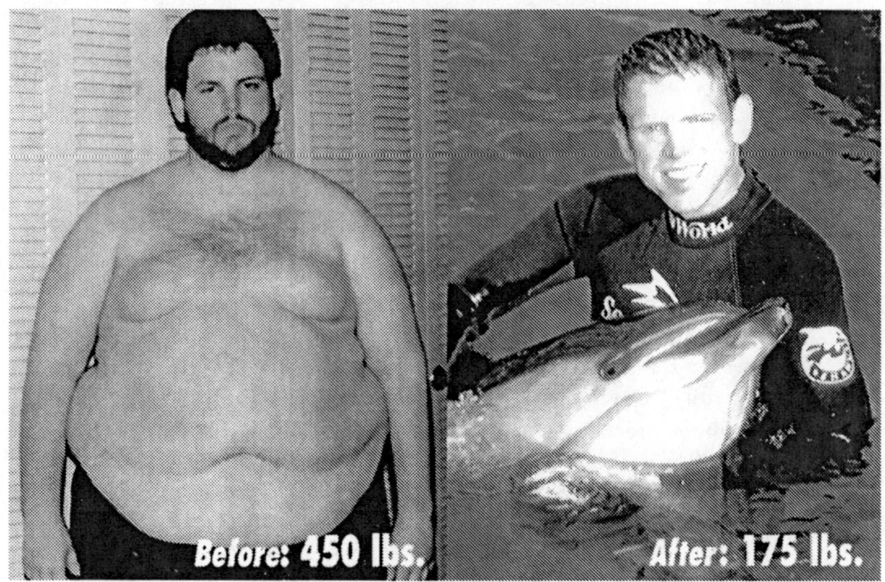

Just Stop Eating So Much!

How it all came to be

Many dieters have said to me, "I would have never guessed you were *ever* fat" – along with "You're so lucky you took off the weight." *Lucky*? *Me*?!

If I'm so lucky, then how do I explain that I was overweight for nearly two decades before I finally *got* lucky? So overweight, in fact, that I couldn't find clothes in my size without special ordering them, broke a movie theater seat on a date, used to pretend to be ordering for a group of people when I was just ordering food to go for myself, and would get completely out of breath just from *talking* to someone on the phone?

Was that the opposite of lucky? No. I was *thinking* and *living* like a fat person.

I realize a lot of overweight people take offense to the word "fat" as a descriptor. But let's not beat around the pudding bowl. Or belly. Or thighs. Or…Well, you get the picture. Fat is where it's at. And it's the *fat mentality* that kept me obese from first grade through college graduation. Sure, I was funny. Sure, I was the life of the party. Sure, I knew how to win friends and influence people. But I was also *fat.* And I had the 60-inch waist to prove it. (*No*, I did not call my belts the rings of Saturn when they circled me.)

Joining different weight loss organizations and self-help groups (even those of the 12-step variety) made me an expert at offering up excuses as to why I couldn't walk up stairs, couldn't fasten my jeans (no button-fly jeans for this tub of lard) and couldn't fly on an airplane without getting a special extension piece for my seatbelt (once again, just imagine the joy in someone's eyes when they see they're going to be crammed up next to a 450-pound man for a six-hour flight).

These organizations offered me *excuses* as to why I was as heavy as I was. It wasn't my fault. The fact that I had extremely abusive parents influenced my eating. I was keeping the world at a distance with my layers of blubber.

And the reason I ate so much? I was searching for love and could only find it in a bag full of Oreos or stacks of potato chips, or maybe a bucket of ribs. Or was it the multiple pizzas washed down with more than one milk shake? Anyway, the point was, I couldn't be held responsible for my massive size because I was a *victim.*

And believe me, I bought into this ridiculous scenario – believing I had no choice but to eat my way to happiness and, therefore, couldn't be held responsible for breaking a wicker chair that I sat in when joining friends for dinner at a Hawaiian-themed restaurant. (Whoever invented wicker furniture obviously had the Olsen twins in mind as houseguests and not someone who made sure McDonald's kept hitting new sales records.)

Anyway, the news was plain and simple. I was an innocent bystander. Halo firmly in place above my head. Angelic wings attached to my back (fat). And sweet, innocent eyes. Blink-Blink.

Get the point, people? Being fat's not my fault!

In reality, these weight loss organizations and self-help groups weren't *helping* me at all. To use their language, they were *enabling* me…giving me excuses for continuing to eat enough food at one sitting to feed a small family of four. The more I saw myself as the victim, the more permission I had to unleash my frustrations onto (or *into*) my belly. And I showed them. Before you could say "Polly, want a cracker?" or "Gregg, want a buffet table?" I was tipping the scales at 450 pounds.

Not that my fancy electronic scale *registered* 450 pounds. I had bought the scale at a doctor's recommendation, since my other scale didn't go above 280 pounds. I was over 300 pounds at the time. The new digital scale would read up to 350 pounds. I knew I'd never hit that. And truthfully, I didn't…I zoomed right past it, to over 450 pounds. I only knew this from buying a doctor's professional digital scale (no truck-weighing highway scales necessary, thank you). When stepping onto my digital scale, post 450 pounds, it would only read "ERR." As mentioned earlier, I'm pretty sure at a certain point the digital read out was "*Get Off*!" when I got *on*.

The fact of the matter is that despite the abuse, the neglect, the traumas of life that we *all* face, I was thinking, eating and *living* like a fat person.

In hindsight, I'm sure these weight loss groups and organizations wanted to *keep* me fat. After all, if I had dropped the pounds under their guidance, I would no longer need to be a member (or a *paying* member, anyway). It never occurred to me, meeting after weekly meeting, that the fact that I and most other members were not losing (and mostly gaining) weight was actually a *benefit* to these groups' bottom line. The fatter we became, the more money they made.

Groups of us who met and became friends at these groups would usually go out after the meeting (and weigh-in) to stuff ourselves at some nearby restaurant. You've never seen an orgy until you've seen a bunch of Weight Watchers members digging into a fried appetizer sampler at TGI Friday's. (Be sure to count all your fingers afterwards - one's likely to have been dipped in sauce and devoured!)

And yet, I continued to pay anyone and everyone who offered a solution, looking for the *cure* to my problems…the book, the pill, the group, the surgery, the *magic formula* that would take me from fat to thin in one fell swoop. But that magic formula never could be found, because it didn't exist. At least not in the places I was looking – and *paying* – for it.

Frustrated, *fat* and out of breath – not to mention stuffed into jeans that were about to put an eye out when the buckle broke loose – I wasn't sure where else to turn. Finally, I found myself considering the last resort – gastric bypass surgery. I'd have a metal ring clamped around my stomach and *that* would cure me once and for all.

Yet as sick (and fat) as I was, I was afraid to have that kind of invasive procedure done to my body. Something deep down inside me knew that wasn't the answer. People were dying as a result of the surgery. And people who had lived were throwing up for weeks after having the procedure, still trying to stuff as much food into their newly small bellies as they could.

I screamed. I shouted. *If this wasn't the cure, then what was*?

I was at my limits – *literally*. Even the big men's clothing stores had only certain sizes they went up to, and I was pushing the boundaries. Wearing (stressing!) a 60-inch waist belt, I was about to start having clothes custom made, or wearing sheets (which I considered, but California King sheets aren't sold in that many places).

I wasn't sure where to turn – or *who to pay* – next. So I approached a colleague at work. He was thin, handsome, athletic and a hit with the ladies. I thought of him as my twin. (Just kidding… At 450+ pounds, I could have been triplets compared to just one of someone his weight.) Anyway, I wondered if perhaps *he* had the magic formula.

We weren't very close. And I wasn't even that comfortable talking to a man about my fat (most members of the weight loss groups and organizations were female). But seeing his chiseled physique and knowing he must have been privy to some sort of secret information that I'd never discovered, I took the risk and decided to let him know I had a weight problem.

Insert long pause here. *As if* he didn't know I had a weight problem (I was 450 pounds, after all)… Like my blocking the sun didn't give him a hint?

He stared at me blankly. Not knowing what to do, I told him about my childhood. About my abusive parents. About all the things that plagued me and *forced* me to start eating and gain weight. (If only I'd already written the "Meet my Belt" section of this book – I could have just handed it to him to read).

His stare continued. I was nervous, anxious…wondering what incredible secret this thin, athletic man who ate anything was going to offer to me. And then, his lips suddenly parted. He prepared to speak. Bright white light seemed to shine down from the heavens! I could hear angels begin to sing! I *knew* I was about to be handed the key to the universe from this insightful Yoda-like creature.

His words? His secret? His key to a life of being thin, fit and happy?

Just stop eating so much!

Huh? No, wait… I wanted real advice, man.

I thanked him, then moved on. I wasn't going to waste any more time with someone who clearly didn't understand the anguish, the pain, the prejudice I was going through in my life. The very reasons that were keeping me fat against my own will.

I shared his callous observation with a few fat girlfriends. Like me, they found his response to be rude, insensitive and crass. They agreed with me. I agreed with them. Then we all finished the ice cream sundaes we were cheating on our diets with.

Weeks went by. The food intake continued. My electronic scale was still reading "ERR." I looked it up in the owner's manual. "ERR" stood for *error* – which the scale registers when weight exceeds 450 pounds. It was official. I was now the size of a small country.

As my food intake continued, so did my obsession with what the "strange" thin man at work had said to me. *Just stop eating so much!* It made no sense. It had no value. No *weight.*

I would see him...Living his life, eating anything he wanted to, fitting into his clothes with ease, winning at romance, enjoying lots of friends... He knew the secret to losing weight and looking great – and yet he wasn't telling *me* what that secret was.

This is when I decided I would play detective and watch him and other healthy, "skinny" people. After all, I'd seen enough cop shows on TV. I'd read enough Sherlock Holmes books while in school (or at least seen a couple of the movies). If this reclusive thin guy wouldn't tell me the secret, I would find out what it was through *secret observation.*

This is when I started to observe the way thin, healthy people (AKA "The Healthies") handle life. The way they think about food. The way they approach living. I actually started keeping notes. Watching what they were doing, what they were eating – how they were *living.*

At the end of the week, I had a pretty interesting list. And now? I'm going to share it with you, so you don't have to secretly stalk your thin, healthy and attractive co-workers or friends.

Stalking the Healthies

- Usually, Healthies *can* eat just one. (They know there's always more if they really want it.)

- Food, self-loathing and clothes being too tight are not subjects that Healthies ever really talk about. They're too busy having fun and living life.

- Bathroom scales do not intimidate Healthies. Nor does any number they see if they step on a scale wreck their day or make them hate themselves.

- When putting food on their plate, Healthies never obsess over how much or how little to serve themselves. Healthies add what they think will be enough, knowing they can always add more later.

- Ice cream and other rich or tempting foods don't occupy the Healthies' mind 24/7. If Healthies are hungry, they eat. If not, they're usually not thinking about food.

- Because Healthies are in touch with their *real hunger*, they know to eat when they feel like it and know to stop eating when they *start* to get full.

- Healthies don't mentally debate whether or not to have dessert hours or even days before they have a meal. They decide during or after the meal and sometimes just have a bite or two without any additional thought.

- When at a party, Healthies don't freak out, thinking that if they have dessert, it will wreck their eating plan and mood or that if they don't have dessert, it will wreck their lives. If they want some dessert, they have some dessert. If not, they don't. Oddly enough, it really *is* that simple.

- It's natural for Healthies to buy rich food, bring the food home, eat just some of the food and then not lay in bed thinking about it. Nor will they get up in the middle of the night and eat the rest while no one's looking.

- Healthies do not think of themselves in terms of "good" or "bad" based on what they've eaten during a particular day or time period.

- Eating is a natural act for Healthies – just like sleeping, talking, laughing or playing. It's just one aspect of life that they don't feel the need to obsess over or talk about ad nauseam.

- Healthies' not only eat nutritious and natural food, they *enjoy* it.

- Taking the stairs, participating in sports or even just taking a walk is something Healthies do regularly. They enjoy how being active feels and therefore do it naturally without much thought.

- Purposely skipping a meal is something Healthies would *never* do.

\+ + + + +

I was both baffled and fascinated by my observations. Sure, it all made sense. But I needed to know *how* these mystical Healthies achieved all of the above.

This is when I started to notice some behavior of my own – along with the behavior of many of my fat friends (AKA "The Heavies"). I figured turn-about was fair play, so I'd do some surreptitious observing and make a list about me and my fellow fatties' habits.

Stalking the Heavies

- Before starting a diet, Heavies indulge in hours or even days of eating, convinced they will never be able to enjoy favorite foods again.

- Self-hatred is a daily (and sometimes hourly) activity for Heavies. Because of this, they often avoid socializing for fear of being adversely judged because of their size. Sadly, it's the Heavies who hate themselves the most.

- Heavies' moods are totally determined by how their eating is going for the day or depending on what number they saw on the bathroom scale.

- If there is food on the plate, Heavies are going to eat it – no matter if they are full, experiencing pain from eating too much or otherwise.

- Food occupies the Heavies' minds 24/7. (I admit this one, *myself* – when I'm having lunch, I'm planning dinner – and sometimes even planning the next day's breakfast!)

- Heavies love trying to trick their bodies when it comes to eating. ("*I'll skip this meal then eat for two at dinner.*") Heavies' bodies never fall for tricks. But Heavies keep trying to come up with new ones.

- Heavies think of chocolate or other rich foods as a seductress that knows no mercy yet that can't be resisted. Similarly, Heavies feel sorry for themselves when it comes to the subject of dessert, thinking it's not fair that they "can't" have it.

- If dessert is being offered, Heavies begin to sweat, panic and freak out – wondering what's going to happen to their world if they have dessert and how they'll survive if they don't.

- Fat-free and other "diet foods" are plentiful in Heavies' kitchen cabinets and refrigerators. These foods are seldom fresh and usually never natural.

- Exercising is not something that Heavies think about – and certainly not something Heavies do. If there's an elevator, escalator or moving sidewalk nearby, Heavies usually take it. Walking, stepping and moving are often avoided.

- Heavies can go all day without eating. But come night-time? *Watch out*!

+ + + + +

Holding these lists side by side, I began to draw some parallels. Or, at the very least, started to make sense of the strange and foreign words my colleague had muttered to me…*Just stop eating so much!*

Suddenly, it was all making sense.

Taking off the weight, getting healthy, and feeling good about myself wasn't about a crash diet, a bottled pill, skipping meals, combining certain food groups, the latest fad diet, deep therapy, surgical procedures or even sewing my mouth shut. It was simply about not eating so much and exercising a little more.

I was stunned. I was shocked.

I immediately wanted to grab for the nearest bag of peanut butter cups.

Yet, I couldn't eat. I was dumbstruck by this simple, yet *pure* advice. It didn't come packaged in some expensive bottle. It was right there before my eyes. And my detective work, comparing the life patterns of Healthies vs. Heavies helped me see the truth.

Taking off the weight was simply about making a life change – a simple life change. It wasn't going to take a lot of thought or a lot of therapy. Nothing like that. It was as simple as changing the channel from The Food Network to ESPN. (From *fat* to *fit*, get it?)

Of course, there was the task of developing healthy eating and exercise plans. I weighed more than 450 pounds. I had to be careful. But more observation and research would soon enlighten me (I'm sharing it all in the following pages of this book – saving you a lot more detective work).

Within weeks, I was following my simple, self-made plan…and the weight was literally *melting off.*

Within a one-year period, I took off more than 250 pounds. (I hate using the word "lost" because it makes it sound like getting thin was an accident, which it wasn't.)

It's so easy, you guys…*Just stop eating so much!*

If I were there with you in person as you're reading this, I'd be grabbing you by the shoulders, gently shaking you, trying desperately to get you to experience the same breakthrough I did.

I know that it's simple advice. But that's because it's *true* advice. And now, because I've done it, because I've taken off more than 250 pounds, because I've *kept it off* for more than 10 years, because I'm healthier and better-looking than I've ever been (yeah, I said it) and because I've been the same *victim* of not only myself, but also the multi-billion dollar diet industry, I'm begging you to realize you're holding the answer to your weight dilemma in your hands.

Together, we're going to conquer this challenge. And it's going to be a lot easier than you think. It's time for change. And that change starts now. Or, I should say, with the very next page…

The Just Stop! Eating Plan

How it works

Following the Just Stop! Plan is easy. That's because you choose 3 meals a day (Breakfast, Lunch and Dinner) from the Just Stop! Menus. It's that simple. Try mixing and matching different meals on different days. Or find a few favorites and stick to those. Just make sure you choose a Breakfast Option for Breakfast Time, A Lunch Option for Lunch Time and Dinner Option for Dinner Time.

Simple, right?

There's also a Snack Options Page for when you really get hungry. But remember: You're supposed *be* a little hungry from time to time. That's because you're goal is to shed your outer later and look and feel your very best. The Just Stop! Eating Plan will take a few days to get used to. But you'll be surprised how easily you adapt to it and how much you look forward to the various meals that are included.

A Splurge Options Page has also been included. This is for special occasions. But this should only be used by people with 20 pounds or less to lose. People who want to take off more than 20 pounds are going to have to toughen up and adapt to the plan. You want to be thin, right? You want to look amazing? You want friends' and family members' jaws to drop when they see you a couple weeks or months from now, right? That's the vision you've got to hold onto.

When all is said and done, it's very simple. You'll be surprised at how simple it is. But that's because losing weight is easy. You just have to make the *simple choice* that you really want a life change and that you're *really* willing to do it. Even if that means cutting back on your food. The whole concept of Just Stop Eating So Much! is based on *not eating so much*. That all begins with you and your commitment to yourself.

Remember, if I can do it, anyone can do it. I believe in you and I know you have what it takes to shed the unwanted weight and be the best you can be.

Today's literally the first day of the rest of your life. Live it to the fullest – while looking and feeling as good as you deserve to.

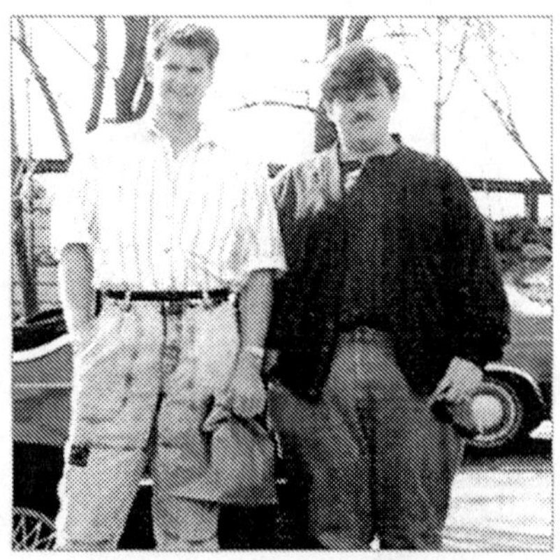

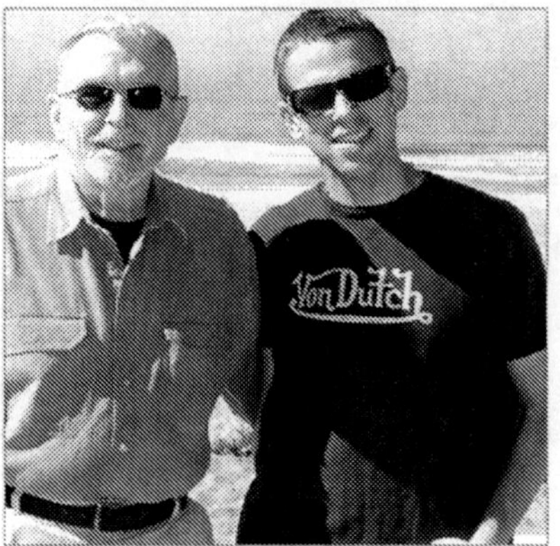
Von Dutch

Just Stop! Meal Guide

First Thing in the Morning

(Well, maybe the *second* thing – but you know what I mean)... Begin every single day with an 8-oz. glass of warm or room temperature water with fresh or organic lemon juice squeezed into it. Not only will this rev up your metabolism and kick it into gear for the day (even before breakfast), it's also a great way to instantly rehydrate after a good night's sleep.

Breakfast Time (Within 1 hour of rising)

Black Coffee or Green Tea (nothing added but water)
The Just Stop Eating So Much! Breakfast Option of Your Choice
A multi-vitamin of your choice

Lunch Time (Midday)

Room Temperature Water or Plain Sparkling Water
The Just Stop Eating So Much! Lunch Option of Your Choice

Dinner Time (At least 4 hours *before* bedtime)

Room Temperature Water or Plain Sparkling Water
The Just Stop Eating So Much! Dinner Option of Your Choice

Snack Time (Midmorning, Mid Afternoon – *only* if needed)

If possible, avoid snacks. But if you're hungry and simply can't wait until your next meal, you're allowed one Just Stop! Snack Option mid-morning and one Just Stop! Snack Option mid-afternoon. No snacking at night whatsoever. After dinner's done, so are you (with eating for the day).

All Day Long

Drink *lots and lots* of room temperature water. Yes, you will likely be in the bathroom a little more than you're used to – but staying hydrated is worth it. As you diet and lose weight, you want to flush out your fat cells and clean out your system. Water is the way to do this effectively and safely. Plus, it helps you stay full. If you're not used to drinking water, get used to it. You want to be thin and gorgeous, right? Then start gulping the water! Your body will thank you for it.

Important Note

If you don't see a food, drink or other edible substance on this plan, you can't have it. (This includes "energy" or "nutrition" bars or any other packaged food that claims to be handy for skipping meals. Skipping meals is *not* good. Real food *is.*) It's simple. Your goal is to transform your body and it's not going to happen by cheating here and there or adding in foods or meal substitutes that aren't part of the plan. The whole idea is to Just Stop Eating So Much! along with eating the *right foods* for your body. And that way of living begins *now*!

Just Stop! Breakfast Options

Just Stop! Breakfast Option #1

1 Slice of Wheat Toast (plain)
1/2 of a large Grapefruit, peeled and sliced into chunks for easy eating

Just Stop! Bonus Tip: Wrap the other half of the grapefruit in cellophane for use for another breakfast later this week.

The wheat bread you choose should have less than 12g of carbohydrates (check the nutrition label). Make sure you avoid white bread at all costs. It does not contain efficient fiber and is metabolized too easily and, therefore, is treated much like sugar in your body. No! Choose healthy wheat bread instead (lightly toasting it enhances its subtle flavors).

Just Stop! Breakfast Option #2

1 Slice of Wheat Toast (plain)
1 medium Orange, peeled and sliced into chunks for easy eating

Just Stop! Bonus Tip: Don't make breakfast a throw-away meal. Take time to arrange the food nicely on the plate and sit down and enjoy your meal – even if you're enjoying it while watching morning news, reading the paper or checking email.

Just Stop! Breakfast Option #3

3/4 cup cooked Brown Rice, served warm, sprinkled with Cinnamon (nothing else!)
1/2 of a medium Banana, sliced into chunks and mixed into the Brown Rice

Just Stop! Bonus Tip: Don't second guess your measuring skills. Get out a measuring cup and measure precisely. You're in control of body and how you look – start exercising that control and never deviate from it.

Just Stop! Breakfast Options (continued)

Just Stop! Breakfast Option #4

1 small Whole Wheat Pita Pocket (plain), sliced open and lightly toasted
1 1/2 cups of fresh Cantaloupe, sliced into chunks

Just Stop! Bonus Tip: When I list a "small pita pocket," I'm referring to a small, normal, reasonably sized pita pocket (not a mini pita pocket or anything like that).

Substitute 1/2 of a medium banana for the Cantaloupe and put the slices into the *un*-toasted Pita with a sprinkle of Cinnamon for a new twist on the Breakfast Sandwich To-Go.

Just Stop! Breakfast Option #5

3/4 cup *dry* Unsweetened Puffed Wheat Cereal (nothing added – not even milk)
1 cup of Sliced Strawberries; mixed into the puffed wheat

Just Stop! Bonus Tip: Puffed wheat cereal is similar to puffed rice. Puffed wheat features a slightly nutty flavor that pairs well with sweetness from the fruit.

The first time you try this mixture (still use a spoon or even a small cocktail fork), you'll think you're crazy for even trying cereal without milk. But this will become a favorite breakfast. You can also try substituting 1/2 of a medium banana for the strawberries for a change in flavor. (The puffed wheat "sticks" to the banana and is delicious!)

Enjoy it with black coffee, green tea or water and learn to savor the different flavors and textures – and remember how much *good* you're doing for your figure.

Just Stop! Breakfast Options (continued)

Just Stop! Breakfast Option #6

3/4 cup of plain oatmeal (cooked, not micro-waved, only adding water)
1 Cup Fresh Raspberries (mixed into the warm oatmeal)

Just Stop! Bonus Tip: Make breakfast a ritual you never skip. Not only is it essential for winning at the *losing game*, it's also usually one time of day you can have to yourself (even if that time of day is before 7am!).

For a change of pace, try substituting 1 cup of fresh blueberries for the raspberries.

Just Stop! Breakfast Option #7

1/2 of a *small* Wheat Bagel, toasted
1 cup of Fresh Pineapple Chunks

Just Stop! Bonus Tip: When I list a "small wheat bagel," I'm referring to a small, normal, reasonably sized bagel (not a mini bagel or anything like that).

And go ahead – get fancy. Nibble at your bagel (make it last) while using a toothpick to serve yourself pineapple chunks. The more you enjoy your meals, the more satisfaction you'll carry into your day.

Just Stop! Lunch Options

Just Stop! Lunch Option #1

Lunch Salad:
6 oz. of Just Stop! 3-Hour Chicken (*See Recipe*), chopped into chunks
Two cups Fresh Cherry Tomatoes, sliced in half
Balsamic Vinegar & Fresh Ground Pepper

Just Stop! Bonus Tip: Prepare enough of the Just Stop! Chicken to last you all week long. The more you prepare ahead, the easier mealtime prep will be.

Just Stop! Lunch Option #2

Lunch Salad:
1 small Fuji Apple, cored and chopped into chunks
1/2 cup Fresh Blueberries
1/2 cup Fresh Raspberries
1/2 cup Fresh Strawberries, Sliced
1/2 cup Lowfat Cottage Cheese
1 tsp. Lowfat Sour Cream
2 tbsp. Chopped Walnuts
Fresh Ground Pepper

Just Stop! Bonus Tip: After tossing the fruit in a bowl, mix the cottage cheese, sour cream, walnuts and ground pepper separately, then add to the top of the fruit mixture.

Limit this lunch option to just *two times* per week (it's a real treat and you'll really crave it!).

Just Stop! Lunch Options (continued)

Just Stop! Lunch Option #3

Lunch Salad:
6 oz. of Just Stop! 3-Hour Chicken (*See Recipe*), chopped into chunks
1 Small Fuji Apple, cored and chopped into chunks
1 cup Fresh Lettuce Mix
Balsamic Vinegar & Fresh Ground Pepper

Just Stop! Bonus Tip: Dump the traditional Iceberg Lettuce and use more flavorful Lettuce Mixes. A favorite of mine is arugula, which offers a rich, almost pepper-like flavor.

Just Stop! Lunch Option #4

6 oz. canned Tuna Fish
Balsamic Vinegar
1 tsp. Organic Lemon Juice
Fresh Ground Pepper
1 cup Fresh Pineapple Chunks
1 cup Fresh Honeydew Melon Chunks

Just Stop! Bonus Tip: Mix the Tuna with the Balsamic Vinegar, Lemon Juice and Ground Pepper the night before and store it in the fridge. The flavors will combine and the tuna will be much more tasty. Serve on the side of your Fruit Salad and enjoy the fresh, healthy flavors.

Just Stop! Lunch Options (continued)

Just Stop! Lunch Option #5

6 oz. of Just Stop! 3-Hour Chicken (*See Recipe*), chopped into chunks
1 Fresh Garden Tomato, sliced into wedges
Fresh Ground Pepper
1 medium Peach, sliced into wedges

Just Stop! Bonus Tip: Arrange everything on the plate, sprinkle the chicken and tomato with ground pepper, then enjoy.

Just Stop! Lunch Option #6

2 cups Raw Baby Spinach Leaves
1/4 cup Lowfat Blue Cheese Chunks
Balsamic Vinegar
Fresh Ground Pepper
2 Slices Swiss Cheese
2 Slices Pepper Jack Cheese (or plain Jack if don't like spicy foods)
1 Slice Wheat Toast

Just Stop! Bonus Tip: Mix the Spinach, Blue Cheese, Balsamic Vinegar and Ground Pepper in a bowl, then serve with the cheese slices and bread on the side. Limit this lunch option to just *one time* per week, due to its rich dairy and higher fat content.

Just Stop! Lunch Options (continued)

Just Stop! Lunch Option #7

2 Eggs, Scrambled (no oil, no nonstick spray – use a Teflon-coated pan)
Fresh Ground Pepper
1 Fresh Zucchini, Sliced
Garlic Powder
Chili Powder
1/2 cup Cottage Cheese

Just Stop! Bonus Tip: Mix the eggs in a bowl with ground pepper before scrambling. While the eggs are cooking, slice the zucchini and place into a microwave safe container with a little filtered water on the bottom. Sprinkle garlic powder and chili powder onto the zucchini, then microwave on high for one minute and allow to steam for a couple more minutes, then drain to serve. This lunch results in a trio of flavors and textures that's hard to beat.

Limit this lunch option to just *two times* per week.

Just Stop! Dinner Options

Just Stop! Dinner Option #1

6 oz. Broiled Steak (seasoned only with Garlic Powder and Ground Pepper)
1 cup Brussels Sprouts (steamed with Garlic Powder and Chili Powder)

Just Stop! Bonus Tip: It's okay to choose a cut of steak with a little fat on it to add to the flavor during the broiling process. But make sure the cut of meat isn't too fatty. Remember when broiling your steak to do so on a nonstick surface. Never use olive oil or nonstick cooking spray of any kind.

You can steam the Brussels Sprouts in the microwave by rinsing them with water, then putting them in a microwave safe container, adding a little filtered water to the bottom and then microwaving them on high (with a unsealed lid on top) for approximately 3 minutes.

Limit this dinner option to just 1 time per week.

Just Stop! Dinner Option #2

Hearty Dinner Salad:
6 oz. of Just Stop! 3-Hour Chicken (*See Recipe*), chopped into chunks
2 cups of Fresh Baby Spinach Leaves
1/2 small Green Pepper, sliced into bite-sized pieces
6 Fresh, Raw Green Beans
Balsamic Vinegar
Fresh Ground Pepper

Just Stop! Bonus Tip: Arrange the chicken chunks on your favorite plate (I like mine cold, from the refrigerator – prepared earlier in the week). Add the spinach on top, followed by the green pepper. Sprinkle with fresh ground pepper, then add Balsamic Vinegar. Arrange the green beans on top, to eat by hand (crunch factor!) as you enjoy the salad.

Just Stop! Dinner Options (continued)

<u>Just Stop! Dinner Option #3</u>

6 oz. Swordfish Steak
Organic Salad Greens
1/2 cup sliced Cherry Tomatoes
1/2 cup sliced Cucumber
Fresh Ground Pepper
Garlic Powder
Balsamic Vinegar

Just Stop! Bonus Tip: Before broiling the Swordfish, sprinkle with Garlic Powder. Then add a few drops of Balsamic Vinegar to the side facing up. Broil the Swordfish on high for 8-10 minutes on each side (using a nonstick surface – no oil or nonstick cooking spray allowed!). When you turn it over, add the Garlic Powder and Balsamic Vinegar to the other side. This will result in a juicy, flavorful piece of fish that's as healthy as it is delicious.

As for the vegetables, mix them together and add pepper and Balsamic Vinegar for the perfect side salad.

<u>Just Stop! Dinner Option #4</u>

Robust Dinner Salad:
6 oz. of Just Stop! 3-Hour Chicken (*See Recipe*), chopped into chunks
2 cups Salad Greens (I prefer Arugula for added flavor and *snap*)
1/2 cup sliced Cherry Tomatoes
1/2 cup sliced Cucumbers
Fresh Ground Pepper
Balsamic Vinegar

Just Stop! Bonus Tip: Arrange the chicken chunks on a dinner plate (I like mine cold, from the refrigerator – prepared earlier in the week). Add the greens on top, followed by the cherry tomatoes and cucumber. Sprinkle with fresh ground pepper, then add Balsamic Vinegar.

Just Stop! Dinner Options (continued)

Just Stop! Dinner Option #5

6 oz. Salmon Steak (with skin, if you prefer)
1 cup Cherry Tomatoes, sliced
Fresh Ground Pepper

Just Stop! Bonus Tip: Talk about simple flavors coming together with hardly any fuss at all! Broil the salmon on high on a nonstick surface (remember: oil and nonstick spray are forbidden!), about 8 minutes each side, depending on the thickness of the cut. The broiler will blacken the skin – making it tasty and flavorful (be careful of small bones, depending on the cut of salmon you've selected from the market).

Once the salmon is ready, plate it. Then pull out a bowl and mix the sliced cherry tomatoes with freshly ground pepper. The cold, flavorful tomatoes paired with the hot, naturally tasty salmon can't be beat!

Just Stop! Dinner Option #6

6 oz. of Just Stop! Chili Chicken (*See Recipe*)
1 cup of fresh Green Beans
1/2 cup Cherry Tomatoes, sliced

Just Stop! Bonus Tip: You'll be surprised how zesty and flavorful this chicken is. I like serving it warm, while serving the vegetables cold (even the green beans). The mixture of textures makes this feel like a special meal – which it is, because it's taking you to your goal of feeling and looking great.

Just Stop! Dinner Options (continued)

Just Stop! Dinner Option #7

6 oz. of lowfat Ground Hamburger Meat
1/2 cup sliced cherry tomatoes
1 cup Brussels Sprouts (steamed with Garlic Powder and Chili Powder)

Just Stop! Bonus Tip: Supermarkets now offer all sorts of healthier options for ground meat. Look for burger meat with 8% fat or less. Then shape the meat into a patty and broil it on high, approximately 5-8 minutes each side, depending on how rare or well done you like your meat. Remember when broiling, do so on a nonstick surface. Never use olive oil or nonstick cooking spray of any kind.

Also, if you prefer not to eat red meat, use ground turkey – just follow the same lowfat guidelines. (By the way, I prefer lowfat to nonfat, because it's more flavorful!)

You can steam the Brussels Sprouts in the microwave by rinsing them with water, then putting them in a microwave safe container, adding a little filtered water to the bottom and then microwaving them on high (with a unsealed lid on top) for approximately 3 minutes. Serve the cherry tomatoes cold and on the side.

Limit this dinner option to just 1 time per week.

Just Stop! Snack Options

(only when absolutely necessary – and only once or twice a day, *if needed*!)

Just Stop! Snack Option #1

1/2 medium cucumber, sliced
Organic Lemon Juice
Ground Pepper

Just Stop! Bonus Tip: Slice the cucumber to resemble potato chips, sprinkle with lemon juice and ground pepper, then enjoy one at a time.

Just Stop! Snack Option #2

Just Stop! Baked Apple:
1 medium Fuji Apple
1/3 cup Organic Lemon Juice
1/3 teaspoon of Vanilla Extract
1/4 teaspoon Cinnamon

Just Stop! Bonus Tip: Core apple, then place in a microwave safe container, sprinkle with lemon juice, vanilla and cinnamon. Cover with plastic wrap, then microwave on high power for approximately 3 minutes. Remove from microwave and let stand for 5 minutes (still covered).

Just Stop! Snack Options (continued)

(only when absolutely necessary – and only once or twice a day, *if needed*!)

Just Stop! Snack Option #3

6 Carrot Sticks
6 Celery Sticks

Just Stop! Bonus Tip: Basic? Yes. Crunchy? Definitely. Enjoy the textures – and get psyched about your decision to transform your body!

Just Stop! Snack Option #4

Cinnamon Banana Surprise:
1 Medium Banana
1 teaspoon of Organic Lemon Juice
1/4 teaspoon Cinnamon

Just Stop! Bonus Tip: Preheat broiler. Split banana in two (length-wise) and place it on a nonstick cooking surface, then onto the broiler rack. Drizzle with lemon juice, sprinkle with cinnamon, lick your fingers (you know you want to), and then broil for 8 minutes, until soft and bubbly.

Just Stop! Splurge Options

(available *only* when you have 20 pounds or less to lose!)

20 pounds or less to lose:	You may choose only 1 Splurge Option for every *two weeks*
10 pounds or less to lose:	You may choose only 1 Splurge Option per week

Just Stop! Splurge Option #1

1 cup of coffee with cream and sugar
Small Wheat Bagel, Sliced, Toasted
With a thin layer of All Natural Peanut Butter

Just Stop! Bonus Tip: "Scoop" out the bulk of the bagel for even less caloric damage during this particular splurge.

Just Stop! Splurge Option #2

1 6-8-oz. glass of Red Wine of Your Choice
3/4 cup of Raw Cashews (plain – no oil, no salt)

Just Stop! Bonus Tip: Finding Raw Cashews (meaning not roasted or salted) is getting easier and easier. They're usually available at organic or whole food-type of markets, but can often be found in "regular" grocery stores, too.

Just Stop! Splurge Options (continued)

(available *only* when you have 20 pounds or less to lose!)

20 pounds or less to lose: You may choose only 1 Splurge Option for every *two weeks*

10 pounds or less to lose: You may choose only 1 Splurge Option per week

Just Stop! Splurge Option #3

1 Splurge Meal at the Restaurant of Your Choice
2 medium glasses of Red Wine

Just Stop! Bonus Tip: Forget whole Splurge (or *cheat*) days or weekends. Those are now a thing of the past. Even just 24 hours of reckless eating can do terrible damage to your Just Stop Eating So Much! Plan. Instead, choose to indulge in one meal. Have whatever you want – but don't eat until you're stuffed. Remember: Once you qualify for the occasional splurge, you can look forward to them and plan for them each week.

Just Stop! Splurge Option #4

1 6-8-oz. glass of Red Wine of Your Choice
1 medium-sized Dark Chocolate Bar (all natural – no additives)

Just Stop! Bonus Tip: Talk about a slice of heaven. Sit back, relax and enjoy the rich taste of decadence. Remember not to overdo it. Enjoy the sensation of the flavors – something you can do without stuffing yourself. And if you choose not drink wine, enjoy 1 cup of coffee (with cream and sugar this one time only, as opposed to drinking the coffee black with nothing else in it).

Just Stop! 3-Hour Chicken Recipe

Ingredients:

1 *huge* package of boneless, skinless chicken thighs
Garlic Powder
Balsamic Vinegar

Preparation:

Use a cast iron pot that can hold as much chicken as you're preparing (I like preparing an extra large package, then using it throughout the week so I don't have to cook it for every single meal I want to use it for).

Place the thighs in the pot, then sprinkle with garlic powder (just on top – no need to make sure every piece gets covered). Then splash on approximately 3-4 tablespoons of Balsamic Vinegar. Put the lid on the pot, then cook on the lowest stovetop flame (or setting) possible for 45 minutes.

After 45 minutes, use oven mitts and the lid to drain *any liquid* out of the pot. Then use a utensil to re-arrange the chicken inside the pot. Next, make sure the lid's in place, place the pot back on the low heat for 30 more minutes.

After 30 minutes, use oven mitts and the lid to drain *any liquid* out of the pot. Then use a utensil to re-arrange the chicken inside the pot. Next, make sure the lid's in place, place the pot back on the low heat for 30 more minutes.

After 30 minutes, use oven mitts and the lid to drain *any liquid* out of the pot. Then use a utensil to re-arrange the chicken inside the pot. Next, make sure the lid's in place, place the pot back on the low heat for 30 more minutes.

Repeat this process until you've reached the 3-hour mark. Then turn off the flame, use oven mitts and the lid to drain *any liquid* out of the pot, and then re-cover the pot and let it sit on the stove to allow the chicken to cool for approximately 30 minutes.

(Double check the chicken to make sure it's cooked through and not pink.) Next, transfer the chicken to a refrigerator safe container and use for your Just Stop! Meal Plans throughout the week.

A note about chicken thighs:

One of my clients asked why I use chicken thighs for this recipe, which are slightly higher in fat grams (about 8.2 fat grams for 6 oz.) than chicken breast (about 6.2 fat grams for 6 oz.). The reason is simple:

Just Stop! 3-Hour Chicken Recipe (continued)

A note about chicken thighs (continued):

flavor. Plus, the only consistent source of fat you're getting on the Just Stop! Plan is from animal protein. And, for the record, 6 oz. of chicken breast has about 284 calories vs. 6 oz. of chicken thighs, which have about 266 calories. So at the end of the day, the difference between the two is negligible. But I find thighs much better for use in the Just Stop! 3-Hour Chicken Recipe.

Just Stop! Bonus Tip: When I store this chicken in the refrigerator, I separate it into 6 oz. serving sizes, making it easy to reach for when it's time to prepare a meal. This chicken is delicious cold. I never re-heat it. But that's always an option, using your microwave.

Just Stop! Chili Chicken Recipe

Ingredients:

6 oz. Boneless, Skinless Chicken Breast
(*or more if you want to prepare extra for use in future meals*)
Crushed Garlic (fresh or from a jar, if packed without oil)
Chili Powder

Preparation:

Place a generous amount of crushed garlic into a bowl - I find cereal bowls work great!

Place several tablespoons of chili powder into a second bowl (a cereal bowl is also a good choice here).

Take chicken out of package and pat dry using a paper towel. Make the chicken as dry as possible, then roll it in the crushed garlic until it's covered. After that, roll it in the chili powder – until the chicken and garlic are covered.

Place this prepared chicken breast into a nonstick frying pan (do not use any oil or cooking spray). Cover the frying pan and place it over low heat. Cook the chicken (covered) for approximately 6-8 minutes. Then uncover the pan, turn over the chicken and cook for approximately 6-8 minutes more, depending on the thickness of the meat. (You want to make sure it cooks through.)

After the chicken is cooked, turn off the heat and let it sit in the covered frying pan for approximately 5 minutes. This adds to the rich flavor as well as the juiciness.

Just Stop! Bonus Tip: Feel free to make more than a single serving. This chicken recipe reheats easily in the microwave (add a droplet or two of filtered water to add back some moisture during the reheating process).

Planning Meals for Families

If you're responsible for fixing meals for other members of your household, don't worry – adapting the Just Stop Eating So Much! meals for people who aren't trying to lose weight is easy. You can basically prepare the same meals, just with a few things added here and there. Do them a favor and follow my guidelines for adding food. This way they'll still be eating healthy and proper portions – which will be as good for them as it is easy for you.

Breakfasts

If you have kids, opt for healthy cereals with fresh fruit and skim milk. For adult members of your household, you can serve the same thing – or even serve Just Stop! Breakfast Options – but add an extra piece of wheat toast when the meal calls for one, or a whole banana if the meal calls for half of one. You can also add a glass of 2% lowfat milk and/or a glass of fresh squeezed (no additives) juice, as well. It's also okay for them to use one normal "pat" of *real* butter. (No substitutes, no fat free, no margarine! Only the "real" stuff so their bodies can process the foods more easily). They can also enjoy lowfat milk and sugar (the *real* thing – no sugar substitutes in their coffee or tea).

Lunches

For kids or adults, it's usually easy to make a sandwich. You can still use the whole wheat bread you use for your meals. Just add a healthy lunch meat (even the 3-Hour Chicken works great) and a small portion of regular mayonnaise (be careful of trans fats and read the label – you want *all natural* ingredients). Better than mayonnaise? Try a Dijon mustard instead. Next, add a piece of fruit and a vegetable. Sugar snap peas make a great lunch addition – they're crunchy, flavorful and easy to eat no matter where you are.

Dinners

This is the easiest meal to adapt for other members of your household. You can basically serve them the exact meal you're having, then simply add a healthy starch to their meal. This can include a baked potato with a small pat of butter, or some brown rice seasoned with garlic powder and pepper. You can also add a tablespoon or two of olive oil to any salads you serve them (in addition to the balsamic vinegar). If they're hearty eaters, offer them a piece of fruit for dessert. You can even serve them sweets from time to time – just make sure they're all natural and don't contain any trans fats. And no matter what weight someone is (whether they need to lose or not), no food should be eaten in excess.

No, it doesn't suck!

Don't feel sorry for yourself when preparing these meals with "extras" for other members of your household. So what if you don't get rice or potatoes? You've made a choice to eat right and *eat less* so you can transform your body. This is a very good thing – so there's nothing to feel sorry about.

Just Stop Eating So Much! Shopping List

FRESH FRUITS
- ☐ Large Grapefruit (*amount* ______)
- ☐ Medium Oranges (*amount* ______)
- ☐ Medium Bananas (*amount* ______)
- ☐ Canteloupe (*amount* ______)
- ☐ Strawberries (*amount* ______)
- ☐ Raspberries (*amount* ______)
- ☐ Pineapple (*amount* ______)
- ☐ Fuji Apples (*amount* ______)
- ☐ Blueberries (*amount* ______)
- ☐ Honeydew Melon (*amount* ______)
- ☐ Peach (*amount* ______)
- ☐ ____________________ (*amount* ______)

FRESH VEGETABLES
- ☐ Cherry Tomatoes (*amount* ______)
- ☐ Garden Tomatoes (*amount* ______)
- ☐ Lettuce Mix (*amount* ______)
- ☐ Arugula Salad Greens (*amount* ______)
- ☐ Baby Spinach Leaves (*amount* ______)
- ☐ Organic Salad Mix (*amount* ______)
- ☐ Green Pepper (*amount* ______)
- ☐ Green Beans (*amount* ______)
- ☐ Brussels Sprouts (*amount* ______)
- ☐ Cucumber (*amount* ______)
- ☐ Zucchini (*amount* ______)
- ☐ Carrot Sticks (*amount* ______)
- ☐ Celery Sticks (*amount* ______)
- ☐ ____________________ (*amount* ______)

DAIRY & EGGS
- ☐ Lowfat Cottage Cheese (*amount* ______)
- ☐ Lowfat Sour Cream (*amount* ______)
- ☐ Lowfat Crumbled Blue Cheese (*amount* ______)
- ☐ Lowfat Sliced Swiss Cheese (*amount* ______)
- ☐ Lowfat Sliced Pepperjack Cheese (*amount* ______)
- ☐ Lowfat Sliced Jack Cheese (*amount* ______)
- ☐ Eggs (*amount* ______)
- ☐ ____________________ (*amount* ______)

BREADS & GRAINS
- ☐ Whole Wheat Bread (*amount* ______)
- ☐ All-Natural Brown Rice (*amount* ______)
- ☐ Small Whole Wheat Pita Pockets (*amount* ______)
- ☐ Puffed Wheat Dry Cereal (*amount* ______)
- ☐ All-Natural Oatmeal (*amount* ______)
- ☐ Small Whole Wheat Bagels (*amount* ______)

SPICES & DRESSINGS
- ☐ Cinnamon (*amount* ______)
- ☐ Vanilla Extract (*amount* ______)
- ☐ Garlic Powder (*amount* ______)
- ☐ Chili Powder (*amount* ______)
- ☐ Peppercorns for ground pepper (*amount* ______)
- ☐ Balsamic Vinegar (*amount* ______)

ESSENTIALS
- ☐ Ground Coffee (*amount* ______)
- ☐ Green Tea (*amount* ______)
- ☐ Organic Lemon Juice (*amount* ______)
- ☐ Chopped Walnuts (*amount* ______)
- ☐ Canned Tuna Fish (*amount* ______)

POULTRY, MEAT & FISH
- ☐ Boneless, Skinless Chicken Thighs (*amount* ______)
- ☐ Boneless, Skinless Chicken Breasts (*amount* ______)
- ☐ Steak (*amount* ______)
- ☐ Lowfat Hamburger Meat (*amount* ______)
- ☐ Lowfat Ground Turkey (*amount* ______)
- ☐ Swordfish Steak (*amount* ______)
- ☐ Salmon Steak (*amount* ______)

OTHER ITEMS
- ☐ ____________________ (*amount* ______)
- ☐ ____________________ (*amount* ______)
- ☐ ____________________ (*amount* ______)
- ☐ ____________________ (*amount* ______)
- ☐ ____________________ (*amount* ______)
- ☐ ____________________ (*amount* ______)

(Make copies of this page so you can use it weekly or whenever you shop)

Notes

What to Expect

The First Couple of Days

Welcome to your life change. I'm not going to candy-coat it. The first couple of days are going to be rough. Your body will not be used to the kinds of food you're eating – or the kinds of portions you're giving it.

You will likely be experiencing a "food hangover" (physical and mental pain from recent binge and junk food eating). You could even experience headaches or extreme sleepiness. This is a result of your body detoxing – getting rid of the crap you've been putting in it for who knows how long. But *stick with it.* Within a couple of days, you're going to be feeling better.

The gross, tired feelings will disappear and suddenly your pants won't be quite so tight and it won't hurt to move and even breathe. You'll realize that you've started something you're committed to – and soon you'll be showing the world that you're really going to do it this time.

You have what it takes. I know you do. So stick with it – no matter what!

Just Stop! Bonus Tip: Most people choose to start diets or new ways of life on a Monday, the beginning of the week. As a "life dieter," I understand this theory. But I suggest you start your Just Stop Eating So Much! Plan on a Saturday. That way you'll have two days to get the headaches, angst, mood swings and lethargy out of the way.

By Monday, you'll have 48 hours of your *new life* under your belt (literally) and will be feeling better, both physically and mentally.

Your Changing Taste Buds

Your taste buds are used to junk food and, quite frankly, *crap* food. Therefore, it's going to take a few days for your tastes to adapt to the pure and natural flavors offered by the healthy foods (and portions) on the Just Stop Eating So Much! Plan. Don't worry.

What might taste bland the first couple of days, will taste better and better the more you wash the crap (and blubber) from your system. Before you know it, you'll be *looking forward* to your Just Stop Eating So Much! meals. They're delicious. They're healthy. And they'll do more than transform your taste buds – they'll transform your life!

What to Expect (continued)

Don't Confuse Hunger for Thirst

Often times, when it *feels* like you're hungry, you're actually thirsty. It's important for people who are taking off excess weight to drink plenty of water – not only to stay hydrated, but also to flush toxins from the body and aid in flushing fat cells of the blubber.

It's important you drink water throughout the day (including before and after working out). Those of you who choose to drink coffee or green tea will need a little more water to balance out the caffeine that's in your system.

No matter what you do, make sure you drink enough water. It's not only important to your success – it's essential.

How Much Water to Drink

Trying to decide how much water is enough water for you? On the average, a person should drink 8-10 eight-ounce glasses of water a day. That's just over 2 quarts. However, it should be noted that someone with weight to lose should consume an additional glass for *every* 25 pounds of excess weight you're carrying. The amount you drink should also increase with brisk exercise or when the weather is hot or dry.

Just Stop! Bonus Tip: Water doesn't have to be boring. Try adding a little organic or fresh squeezed lemon juice to filtered water for a little more flavor. You can also drink sparkling water. Just make sure it has no additives (some seltzers have sodium).

Also, when you're drinking enough water, you're going to be using the restroom frequently. This is actually very healthy. Just make sure you plan your water drinking for times when you'll be nearby an easy-to-access bathroom.

Spa Water Recipe

You can also make something I call **Spa Water**, which has become a favorite of friends who visit me. Take a pitcher of filtered water, then add 10 fresh cucumber slices. Next cut a washed lemon into wedges and squeeze the juice into the pitcher, then add the squeezed lemon wedge. Cover the pitcher and let it sit in the fridge for about 24 hours. The resulting water will be crisp, cool and flavorful – a real pick-me-up and even somewhat of a treat. Serve over ice with a fresh-cut lemon wedge on the glass as a garnish.

What to Expect (continued)

More Good Reasons to Drink Lots of Water

- Water is a natural appetite suppressant and helps your body metabolize stored fat
- Water helps maintain proper muscle tone
- Water helps skin look radiant
- Water helps relieve constipation and helps rid your body of waste
- Drinking enough water is the best way to fight fluid retention or bloating

Go Gourmet – You Deserve it

Be sure to savor the flavor! Since Balsamic Vinegar and Ground Pepper are two staples for adding some oomph to your meals, go ahead and treat yourself.

Buy one of the finer balsamic vinegars, not just the generic store brand. And get yourself a pepper mill and enjoy fresh ground pepper on your food. You'll be surprised how robust the flavor is compared to "average pepper." It makes a difference, trust me!

Just Stop! Bonus Tip: Beware the Balsamic! Sure, it's flavorful. Sure, it's your answer to salad dressing on the Just Stop! Plan. But it's also extremely easy to spill (or splash!) and stains just about anything it comes into contact with.

I jokingly call Balsamic Vinegar "Acid," because that's what you would think it was based on my reaction to a balsamic spill. And that's because I know it stains things in an instant. (If it does spill, I suggest quickly soaking it up with a paper towel and sparkling water.)

So be extra cautious when preparing meals with it and even when eating it!

What to Expect (continued)

Don't Make *Your* Business Everyone Else's Business

If you're like me, when starting a new diet or exercise plan in the past, you've trumpeted it to the rest of the world. Or at least people you come across in your every day life. Even though, really, it's none of their business. This time, why not *keep it to yourself*?

You don't have to broadcast *your business* to other people. You're making a simple, quiet, productive choice that is going to enhance the every aspect of your life. Sure, people are going to eventually notice you're looking better, feeling better and smiling more. But let them notice it and say something (that's *so* rewarding) instead of you letting them know "Hey, look at me – I'm on a diet."

Also, you want to spend less time *thinking* about what you're doing, as well. Don't overanalyze it in your head, constantly debate it or over-think it. You've made the choice. Now do it. By making your life changing decision a more "quiet one," it becomes more personal and much more *real*. This is about you doing something for you. Again, it's no one else's business. Even though eventually people in your life (even mild acquaintances) *will* ask you what you're doing differently in your life, because they're not going to be able to keep from noticing how amazing you're looking. And that's because you *are* amazing. Believe it – 'cause it's true.

Maintain an Organized Kitchen

Once again, I'm not going to lie to you. The first couple of days and even the first week can be tough. You are changing old habits and eating new foods. One of the keys to success will be keeping an organized kitchen. This means planning out your meals, shopping for ingredients and organizing your kitchen *before* you actually start the Just Stop! Plan. (See the easy-to-use Shopping List on Page 49.)

Depending on your level of will power, you won't necessarily want to go to the grocery store during your first couple of days on the plan and see foods that you find tempting. Instead, buy your Just Stop! Ingredients before your begin the plan and have them on hand. I suggest filling out the Food Diary (page 75) for the week ahead, then completing your Shopping List. This way you'll know exactly what you'll require, food-wise, for the upcoming week. Have your kitchen prepared for this new choice and your new lifestyle. Reorganize your refrigerator and have it ready to serve *your* needs on the Just Stop! Plan. Keeping an organized kitchen really *will* make a helpful difference to your success.

What to Expect
(continued)

Maintain an Organized Life

Speaking of organized kitchens (see previous page), you'll also want to keep an organized life.

This extends outside of the kitchen – into the rest of your home and even the way you conduct yourself from day to day. Think about your home, your life (work, rest and play) and make a commitment to being more organized with your time. Take a moment every evening to think about what you want to accomplish the next day. Make a few notes – even create a to-do list or two.

It will really help to keep everything in your life running as smoothly as possible, so when "little surprises" do occur, they don't throw you off – either mentally or (just as bad) eating-wise.

I love making what I call **A-B-C Lists**. These keep me from getting overwhelmed with all I have to do (which can "shut me down," mentally). Keep a notebook, pad of paper or small journal handy at all times. And use 3 pages to create an A List, a B List and a C List.

(I prefer writing things down instead of programming them into my PDA, but if that works for you, keep the lists electronically.)

> **For A Tasks**, list things you *must* accomplish during that particular day.
>
> **For B Tasks**, list things that are secondary, but still important and that need to be taken care of.
>
> **For C Tasks**, list things that don't necessarily need to be done that particular day, but that you want to keep on your to-do horizon (and not forget about).

You'll find that the more organized you are, the more you'll accomplish. The more you accomplish, the better you'll feel about yourself – and that will extend to your Just Stop! Success. No kidding!

What to Expect (continued)

Sleep Tight

Make sure you schedule enough time for enough sleep – 7 to 8 hours *at least*! Your body is going through amazing changes on this plan, and it needs its rest to achieve desired results. I know we all lead busy lives and it's easy to "steal time" from bedtime. But you're only hurting yourself when you do this.

Getting enough sleep is essential to your success. Think of a good night's sleep as "Beauty Rest" (*literally*!) and enjoy it for all its worth. The web contains lots of helpful articles on sleep as it relates to weight loss. You also might find this link helpful:

http://www.helpguide.org/life/sleeping.htm

Eating "Clean"

As you enjoy the foods, meals and portions offered on the Just Stop Eating So Much! Plan, you'll also find your body and metabolism are changing for the better. Part of the reason for this, is the removal of chemicals, trans fats and other dangerous substances often found in mass-produced food. Even packaged foods in so called natural and "whole food" type of markets are loaded with sodium to enhance flavor.

Be careful of anything packaged (cold, frozen or room temperature) that has a long shelf life. These types of foods contain preservatives and other additives that aren't healthy for your body.

Also be aware of "diet foods" marketed directly toward those of us who are trying to be healthy. Just because it has a green package (the food industry's "signal" that this is a "healthier" choice), doesn't mean it's healthy for you. The fresher, more natural and more pure your food is, the easier your body can process it and the more effective your metabolism will be.

The incredible amounts of salt and man-made chemicals used to "enhance" food are poison to your system. Your body doesn't know how to process these unnatural additives. You'll discover you feel better and look better if you eat food that is fresh and pure (without any chemicals or additives).

This new look won't just be limited to your body size. Your skin will glow. Your hair will look healthier. And how you're *feeling* will improve vastly, as well.

What to Expect (continued)

Just Stop! Bonus Tip: Do yourself a favor and become more aware of dangerous food additives. You can do your own online research. But I suggest starting with these websites for helpful information:

http://bantransfats.com/

http://www.dh.gov.uk/en/index.htm

http://www.ffts.com/loso.htm

http://www.cfsan.fda.gov/~dms/foodlab.html

The Just Stop! *Do* List

- Eat at regular intervals. In other words, have your meals at approximately the same time every day.

- Only eat grain-based carbs as outlined in the Just Stop! Breakfast – and occasionally Lunch – Options.

- Don't skip out on anything listed in the meal plans. Even though you want to Just Stop Eating So Much!, you also want to feed your body the necessary nutrients it needs to give you energy as well as to provide your metabolism with what it needs to whittle you down to that sexy beast waiting to be discovered underneath your "outer layer".

- If you're a red meat eater, limit those meal options to just two Just Stop Eating So Much! Dinner Options each week.

- Whenever possible, avoid canned or processed fruits or vegetables. You want them to be as fresh as possible – even organic if your market offers that option. Always wash fruits and vegetables thoroughly, then slice them or prepare them just before eating, so they pack as many nutrients as possible. Remember, you want to be as healthy on the *inside* of your body as you're going to *look* on the outside.

- Drink lots of water throughout the day. The extra trips to the bathroom will be worth it. Flush those fat cells and get sexy!

- Avoid snacks whenever possible. But when you must indulge, only have one of the Just Stop Eating So Much! Snack Options.

- Season foods only with pepper, balsamic vinegar or the few spices offered in the Just Stop Eating So Much! Meal Options and recipes. Never add any salt or oil to your food. (Your body will get the fat it needs from the fat that is naturally present in the protein you're eating – you don't need any additional oil! Not even "healthy" olive oil!)

- Incorporate exercise into your Just Stop Eating So Much! Plan. Get moving for at least 30 minutes, four to five times each week. Gauge the activity based on your current physical health, then increase it as necessary. If you're unsure of what's safe, ask your physician or a local exercise professional (such as a trainer at a local gym – just pay for one session and get all the tips!)

The Just Stop! *Don't* List

- Avoid eating any additional fat. It can be found naturally in some of the foods in the Just Stop Eating So Much! Meal Options. Other than that, skip it: olive oil, cooking oil, even non-fat cooking sprays are all forbidden. You want to shed the weight, not make it more difficult to do so. You're going to get the "fat" you need from the protein you're eating. *No added fat whatsoever!*

- Never have sugar, sweets or candy of any kind.

- Don't use any artificial sweeteners or fat substitutes. If it's not natural, you're not putting it in your mouth (much less your body).

- Be careful not to consume too many cups of black coffee or even green tea. Both have caffeine and can make you jumpy and make it more difficult to go to sleep at night. As a general rule, I suggest not consuming any caffeinated drinks after 12 noon. That way your body has time to metabolize the caffeine before bedtime.

- Stay away from sodas – even diet sodas! Instead, enjoy room temperature water (filtered or bottled) or sparkling water (make water your preferred drink during meals).

- This should go without saying, but just to be clear: Never consume anything fried or that is smothered in a cream sauce.

- Don't drink any alcoholic drinks if you have more than 10 pounds to lose. When you're within 10 pounds of your goal weight, you can add 2 to 3 glasses of red wine *per week* to the plan (note: that's per week, not per day).

- Avoid salt at all costs. *Never* add it to anything you prepare or eat.

- Don't eat dinner too close to bedtime. Schedule your last meal so you're finished eating at least four hours before you go to bed.

- Never skip meals. Especially breakfast. Most "lifetime dieters" I know skip breakfast – then wonder why they "Do fine during the day, but then end up bingeing and cheating at night." *Um, hello*? It's because you're not giving your body what it needs at the beginning of the day. Think about the *word* 'Breakfast' – as in Break Fast (you are *breaking* the *fasting* cycle you've put your body through overnight while not eating for 8-12 hours). Breakfast is essential for kick-starting your metabolism and providing your body with what it needs to succeed in every aspect of your life (including shedding the blubber)!

The Just Stop! Dining Out Guide

Here's the deal…If you have 20 pounds or more to lose, I suggest skipping on the dining out altogether. I know that's a drag. And I can hear you moaning about special occasions or important business lunches.

Whatever.

Do you want to be thin, or not? I took off more than 250 pounds in less than a year – and it didn't happen by making excuses as to why I "needed" to go to a restaurant and eat away from home or eat food I hadn't prepared myself.

This is where you prove to yourself that you're really committed to making a lasting and positive change in your life. In order to accomplish this amazing feat, you're going to have to make some sacrifices. That means eating less and not eating out – even if you have to skip the occasional special function.

Commit to yourself. Your body, your mind, your health are all worth it. And the people in your life who really matter are going to understand why you have to cut back from socializing.

People may balk a little. But when they see that you're *really doing it* this time, they're going to have a newfound respect for you and start making plans that don't revolve around restaurants or party food. You have to remember what's important here: *You*. Period.

Other people will have to understand. And, more important, *you* will have to understand. Accomplishing this goal is going to take some sacrifice. And this is one of those times.

If you absolutely *must eat out* (and I don't really buy that, by the way), here are a few tips for helping you avoid wrecking what you've worked so hard to accomplish:

- Avoid fats at all cost! (This is tough in a restaurant, because fat and salt are added to just about everything. Ask any gourmet chef what ingredient they use the most and they will tell you "Butter." No kidding!)

- Avoid starches. They aren't as easy to spot on a menu. But stay away from breads, pastas, potatoes and rice and you'll be making good headway.

The Just Stop! Dining Out Guide (continued)

Dining Tips (continued from last page):

- If ordering a salad, request vinegar on the side (many places offer balsamic vinegar now, so ask for that by name). Remember: No olive oil. No! No! No!
- Ask that any vegetables be steamed with no oil, butter or salt added.
- When ordering meat, seafood or poultry, look for these descriptions: boiled, broiled (ask for dry-broiled), grilled, poached or steamed.
- No matter what, avoid any foods that contain these descriptors: creamed, fried, sauce, marinated, sautéed, scalloped, smoked, tempura or teriyaki.

Just Stop! Exercise Guide

Get Moving!

An essential part of your Just Stop Eating So Much! success is exercise. Got that? It's not an *optional* part of the plan. It's a must! By moving your body, you're kick-starting your metabolism, burning fat and building muscle.

What's more, you're going to be improving your inner health – heart, organs, muscles, joints – you name it. There's no excuse not to exercise – no matter what your fitness level.

The key is being *smart* about exercise. This means doing what's reasonable for your current body type and your current state of health. You don't want to hurt yourself or be in too much pain.

Exercising should be fun. Not only will it increase your energy, it will cause endorphins to surge throughout your body, which dramatically improves your mood (think of it as nature's antidepressant).

Exercise can also help balance out your metabolism. If you're anything like me, you've started and stopped lots of different diets over and over. This can really screw up your natural metabolism and make your whole "system" slow down. Exercise helps kick this system back into gear. It helps your body function better on all levels.

And the best part? Exercise does as much for your outward appearance as it does for your internal health. There's nothing wrong with letting your vanity fuel your efforts. You know you're a hot, sexy thang just waiting to be discovered. Exercise is going to help uncover that beast sooner rather than later.

When you're exercising in conjunction with your Just Stop Eating So Much! Meal Plan, you're doubling your efforts and speeding up your results. If you have to, start slow (and safe). But definitely *start*…today!

Posture is Everything!

Make sure that you don't live life in a slump – whether you're working at your desk, cooking in the kitchen, running an errand or exercising. Stand up tall, pull your shoulders back, suck in that tummy and keep your head held high (imagine carrying a stack of books on the top of it).

Making sure you keep proper posture during exercise and all other tasks of daily living will not only increase exercise's effectiveness, it will also improve your overall health and appearance.

Just Stop! Exercise Guide (continued)

Walk the Walk:

The best exercise for every fitness level is also the easiest to do: walking. That's right… Good old-fashioned walking. The key is to walk with proper posture (see "Posture is Everything," on the previous page) and to pump your arms back and forth while taking steps. Those at lower fitness levels can pace themselves and start out slowly. Even just 10 minutes, 4 days a week will be beneficial. Then *add* to those 10 minute sessions each week.

Make sure you always suck your stomach in while you walk. Think of using the muscles you'd use if you were trying not to pee. You want to work those muscles constantly. If you walk with proper posture and suck in your stomach the whole time, you will not only burn calories, but also work your abdominal muscles. (And don't forget to pump those arms!)

You're not out taking a casual stroll. You're working that body and working it hard. Try and work up to a pace that will cause you to break a sweat. You want to work hard, not soft. Use the time for what it's meant for: transforming your body.

Soon, you can be power walking 45-60 minutes each time you work out, and making a huge difference in your weight loss efforts. The best part is that you don't need a treadmill or even a gym membership to enjoy the benefits of walking.

Walk around your neighborhood (keep moving in place when you reach a traffic light and have to wait to cross the street). Of course, you can also drive to a local park or, better yet, a hiking trail that offers hills (great for the legs and butt). And if the weather's rainy or cold, get your butt to the mall. Senior citizens have been doing mall walks for years – and it's dramatically improved their health. You can do the same thing – no matter what age you're at.

Walking is an amazing workout. Make sure you're dressed properly for the weather (including a pair of comfortable and supportive walking shoes or sneakers) and get moving!

For those of you who *do* happen to belong to a gym and/or own a treadmill, treadmills can be great "partners" for your walking workout. Try setting the incline higher than level and walk with speed up a simulated hill. But *never* try to hold onto the machine. You will see people at the gym reading magazines, holding on or walking and talking. No! No! No!

Just Stop! Exercise Guide (continued)

Walk the Walk (continued from last page):

You are there to work out. Pump your arms, suck in your stomach, breathe properly and work that body. You're not there to socialize or show someone your new workout clothes. You're there to transform your body! So do it!

Workout Partners

Working out with a buddy is a fun and helpful thing to do. You can both motivate one another. But if your friend isn't able to make your workout date, still get out there on your own. There are no excuses for not moving and exercising. Sometimes the best workout partner comes in the form of an iPod or MP3 player. Put your favorite music on there and create a playlist of songs that get you moving. Then strut your stuff to the beat. You can do it!

Muscle Training

It's important to incorporate resistance training (weightlifting, etc.) into your workouts. By adding resistance training to your routine, you'll build up muscle mass. This will result in not just looking better (and *hotter*), but also in your body starting to burn more calories, more often. Muscle mass requires more internal fuel to maintain than non-muscle mass - meaning that people with defined muscles burn more calories even when they're sleeping. There are other great reasons to have muscle mass in your body, too. It makes you stronger, healthier and more confident. You can purchase your own hand weights from sports supply stores or even join a gym when you're ready to do so. Yes, a gym membership costs money – but you're worth it!

The Fountain of Youth

One of the most powerful additions I've made to my own exercise program is the practice of **yoga**. I was resistant to it at first. It was challenging for me to quiet my mind and go through the paces with the rest of the class. But soon I learned to love yoga for its mind-transforming benefits as well as its benefits for my body and even internal organs.

But even more than that, I found nothing transformed my formerly fat body into a leaner, sexier and more defined one like yoga. Even after years of other forms of exercise, I found yoga's benefits could be seen almost immediately. Classes for every level are available – both at gyms, community centers and even on DVD (rent a couple until you find one that works for you, then buy that one).

Just Stop! Exercise Guide (continued)

The Fountain of Youth (continued):

When you look around a yoga class, you'll be amazed at the different ages of the students. I'm always impressed and inspired by people in their 60s and 70s who are able to do poses more elegantly and athletically than I can. They look amazing, too – their skin, hair and body shape are pure inspiration. Yoga is as good for you internally as it is for you externally. And your mind and spirit benefit, too. I suggest adding yoga to every exercise program. It will literally transform your life. For more information, try surfing the web to these or other yoga-related addresses:

http://www.holisticonline.com/Yoga/hol_yoga_intr.htm

http://www.yogasite.com/yogafaq.html

http://www.yogasite.com/postures.html

Two important words in regard to working out: *No Excuses*!

When I was taking off more than 250 pounds, I was working full time in New York City while living in New Jersey. I had a 90-minute commute each way, and was expected to be at the office for about 10 hours. This meant I was away from home for 13 hours – yet I still found time to work out.

I'm not showing off. I'm just letting you know there are no excuses for not working out. I don't care how busy you are. If you're *really committed* to this change, then you're going to find time. It might be when the kids are finally asleep. It might be at the crack of dawn – or *before* the crack of dawn.

Presently, I live in Los Angeles and get up at 4:30 every *morning* to exercise – even though I'm running my own business, which requires my attention 24/7. When you're committed, you make time. You find time. You do what you have to do. And you *should* be committed. After all, we're talking about an amazing change for your body, your health and your life.

No excuses! Exercise 3 to 4 times a week. It's essential!

Just Stop! Exercise Guide (continued)

Exercise for Every Level

On the following pages, you'll find a series of 8 exercises that most fitness levels can accomplish without too much strain and effort (adapt the exercises when necessary, and I encourage you to check with your health professional before starting any exercise regimen). Remember to take it easy the first time you attempt it. After you get used to it, you'll find this regimen can really work to change your body structure. Do this routine for about an hour, at least three times per week (four is ideal). Eventually not only will you warm up to it, you'll also begin to like it!

Before the workout:

Be sure to warm up for approximately 10 minutes before beginning the workout (walking from a slow pace to a quick pace can be a great warm up – along with easy movements like toe touches and side bends).

During the workout:

Breathing slowly and at an even pace is essential. Try and breathe in through your nose, out through your mouth. Make sure you get your heart rate going and that you sweat. You want to tax your body and burn lots of calories while building up muscle and stamina!

After the workout:

Be sure and cool down to prevent any cramping or soreness (caused by blood concentrates in the muscles and accumulating lactic acid). Roll your shoulders and head slowly. Shake out your arms and legs and stretch in the same way you did during the warm up.

The Exclusive Just Stop! Workout

No Gym Required!

Step 1: Warm up time: Toe touches might seem old fashioned – but they're a great warm-up. Stand straight with feet shoulder width apart, arms over your head. With a slight bend in your knees, reach down with your right hand and touch your left foot (or get as close to it as possible without straining your lower back). Return to starting position, then touch your left hand to your right foot.

Alternate in each direction about 10 times.

Step 2: Cardio time: To build up your cardiovascular fitness, start with a vigorous walk. Slowly build to a light jog and eventually to a three mile run for a 30-minute interval. Be cognizant of your current fitness level and current weight. You don't want to damage your knees or joints. As you progress and your endurance increases and overall health improves, you'll want to work up to 45 or even 60 minutes of cardio. You want to sweat and move and feel like you're *really* working out. Change it out for more variety – you can alternate power walking with running (careful of your knees!), cycling, jumping rope or even swimming to change things out. (Changing things out is very important to any fitness regime).

The more you keep your body "guessing," the faster it's going to change!)

Step 3: Ab time: Let's do sit-ups! Lie on your back with knees bent and your feet flat on the floor. Clasp your hands behind your head and bring your left elbow to your right knee while also tilting your pelvis upward and curling your upper body forward (toward the knee). Think of "pressing down" (internally) against your stomach (the same sensation as if you're trying *not* to urinate!). Hold for 5 seconds, then lower to starting position and repeat on the opposite side.

Work up to 3 sets of 25 repetitions.

Step 4: More abs, more *fab*: Crunch time, people! Lie on your back with your legs straight ahead and your arms at your sides. Lift your right leg straight to the ceiling and left leg a foot off the floor. Tilt your pelvis and internally "suck in" your stomach (same "trying to stop the pee" sensation). Bring your head toward the right knee and hold for 5 seconds. Return to starting position, then repeat on the opposite side. Pay attention to your lower back, which will also strengthen as a result of this exercise.

Do 3 sets of 10 repetitions.

(continued on the next page)

The Exclusive Just Stop! Workout (continued)

Step 5: Let's ride a bike (without the bike): Lie on your back with arms straight at your sides, palms facing down. Lift your legs and lower back off of the floor, toward the ceiling. Move legs up and down (sort of in a circular fashion, as if you're riding an imaginary bicycle).

Continue for 2-5 minutes.

Step 6: Make your stomach stunning: Rollovers are a great way to increase your core strength. Lie on your back, with legs straight ahead and both arms on the floor. Raise your legs to 90 degrees without bending your knees. Slowly lower legs to the right, *without* touching your feet to the floor and while keeping your shoulders flat to the floor. Bring legs back to the center, then lower to the opposite side.

Do 3 sets of 10 reps (each side).

Step 7: Push-up time: Lie face-down on the floor, with hands shoulder-width apart, flat on the floor, shoulder-length apart, fingers pointing forward. Supporting your body weight with your hands and the balls of your feet, straighten your arms without locking your elbows (always keep a slight bend to prevent strain). Legs should remain straight, with knees and feet together. Bend elbows (keeping them close to your body) and lower your body until *just before* your chest touches the floor, then come back up again.

Try starting with 2 sets of 20 repetitions, eventually working up to a third, fourth and even a fifth set. (You can do it!)

Step 8: Cool down time: Start with hamstring stretches like this one. Stand straight with your feet about shoulder-width apart. On the balls of your feet, rotate feet and body to the right. Next, lean forward on your right foot by bending at the knee. Keep your left leg straight back and weight on the ball of your foot. Hold for 30 seconds, then return to starting position.

Do each side at least 3-5 times.

The Exclusive Just Stop! Workout (continued)

Just Stop! Bonus Tip: Successful exercise and day-to-day living are both about having a strong core. You'll find this principle is taught in properly-instructed yoga classes. But it's a concept you can put to work every day, every *hour* – and especially during exercise. *Always* hold your stomach in and work your core abdominal muscles. Not only will this provide strength and increase endurance, it will also help you protect your lower back and other joints and ligaments while you workout.

You should also hold in your stomach during all aspects of daily living – sitting at the computer, cooking in the kitchen, even when watching TV. Sure, relax your stomach when you're in the bathtub or going to bed. But otherwise, suck in those abs. Not only will your posture, health and strength improve, but you'll also transform your body.

Nothing's as *sexy* as a flat, toned stomach. And you're going to have one! I know you can do it. *I believe in you*!

Motivating Reasons to Workout

Looking Good
Regular exercise helps you take off weight by burning calories and raising your metabolic rate. Yeah, I know you knew this. But sometimes it helps to see it in print. And the best part? Even when your workout's through, you'll keep burning calories while resting because your metabolic rate remains elevated several hours after working out.

Feeling Good
Exercise helps alleviate tension and makes you feel great. In fact, hormones excreted during exercise can help you not only relieve stress, but also help with depression.

Inside Out
Numerous medical studies document that exercise helps lower cholesterol by reducing blood lipid levels. Plus, exercise helps blood circulation improve, which can help deliver more oxygen to each of your cells. Exercise also helps bodies retain more calcium – important for anyone getting older (that's all of us, people – but we don't have to *look* like we're getting older!).

Breath of Life
When you exercise, you breathe more deeply and regularly – causing your lungs to work more efficiently. That means next time you climb a flight of stairs or run for a Frisbee, you'll be less winded.

Impressive Results
Exercise can help build your self-confidence and self worth. You're setting goals, achieving them and seeing amazing results as part of the process. This helps you realize you're in control of your life – and that you can accomplish anything you set your mind to.

Think Again
Regular exercise can improve your thought processes. Physical activity actually results in you thinking more clearly and concentrating more easily throughout the day (not just when working out).

Express Yourself
Different exercises offer something for everyone – no matter what kind of mood you're in. Feel like being alone? Try swimming, hiking or taking a walk. Want to join a group? Attend an aerobics or yoga class. Do what feels good to you. Just make sure you *do* the do!

Tracking Your Just Stop! Success

The day you begin your diet, you need to weigh and keep track of that weight. The number might be frightening. But remember: It's just a number. And if you stick with the Just Stop! Plan, that number will be part of your permanent history in a matter of days.

You will be tempted to weigh more often, but take my advice! You should weigh only *once a week, first thing in the morning* (*after* using the bathroom but *before* your lemon water). For accurate weighing, I suggest purchasing an electronic scale with a lithium battery (they never wear out). That way you have an accurate "read" of your body weight each time you weigh.

Also, *never* weigh on any other scale – ever! Only track your success on *your* scale, once a week. Even if you have a medical appointment and they want to weigh you as part of the procedure, tell them you don't want to know your weight and for them to keep it to themselves. Then keep your eyes closed while you're on the scale. This might seem like a small detail, but you don't want anything to throw off your success. And different scales are going to register different weights – no matter how accurate they are.

Use the **Just Stop Eating So Much! Success Tracker** on page 73 to track your success on the program. You'll see a place to fill in the date, followed by your weight, your measurements and even your percentage of body fat. After all, weight loss is just one part of your success. That's why measuring your body parts once a week is a great idea, as well.

And calculating your body fat percentage doesn't require calipers, an expensive scale or a visit to a medical professional. Instead, check out the website below, which offers a pretty accurate body fat percentage estimate based on information you fill in each time you visit:

http://www.healthcentral.com/cholesterol/home-body-fat-test-2774-143.html

Even more important than measurements of any kind is how you look and feel – along with the health benefits. I encourage you to take pictures of yourself along the way. (I took one of myself after every time I weighed – usually once a week – many of which are featured on page 7.)

Speaking of pictures, you might be wondering why this book is full of Before and After pictures of me. It's not *just* because I'm fun to look at (I'm kidding – *sort of*), but because I want to inspire you. I've been on "the other side." I know what it's like to have people stare at my size in horror, wondering where I managed to find clothing big enough to fit my body. And now? I'm considered "thin and normal" by society's standards. I took this amazing journey

Tracking Your Just Stop! Success (continued)

and succeeded. And I'm here to remind you: If I can do it, anyone can do it. That's why I'm sharing the pictures – as added inspiration.

Too often so-called "weight loss gurus" don't have "Before and After"-style pictures because they really haven't taken the journey. I have. And the pictures are proof.

I encourage you to take lots of pictures of your journey, as well. They will be a testament to your progress, your willpower, your success. (And I hope you'll *share* your pictures with me, too!)

As you watch yourself transform in the pictures, think about being able to wear any kind of clothes you want to… about being able to be active without being out of breath…about walking into a room and overhearing people commenting on your smile instead of your girth.

You'll also find a **Just Stop Eating So Much! Food Diary** on page 75. You can make copies of this page and use it to write down *everything* you eat. (I fill out mine *before* I use the Shopping List on page 49 to shop for the week – so I know just what I'll need.) Keeping a log of your food intake (including portions) will help you stay on the plan. By tracking everything you put in your mouth, you'll become more aware of your eating – and more aware of the amazing choice you have made for your body and your life. You *can* do this!

Just Stop! Bonus Tip: One of my clients in Tennessee makes copies of the Shopping List, Success Tracker and Food Diary on 3 different colors of paper and keeps them in a colorful binder for easy organization while keeping track of her incredible success.

Just Stop Eating So Much! Success Tracker

date	weight	body fat%	chest	right arm	left arm	waist	hips	right thigh	left thigh

(Make copies of this page so you can use it until you reach your goal)

Notes

Just Stop Eating So Much! Food Diary

Week Of________________

SATURDAY

Breakfast: *Just Stop Breakfast Option* _____
Lunch: *Just Stop Lunch Option* _____
Dinner: *Just Stop Dinner Option* _____
Snack: *Just Stop Snack Option* _____ *(only when absolutely necessary, see Snack Options page)*
Splurge: *Just Stop Splurge Option* _____ (only if you have less than 20 pounds to lose, see Splurge Options page)

SUNDAY

Breakfast: *Just Stop Breakfast Option* _____
Lunch: *Just Stop Lunch Option* _____
Dinner: *Just Stop Dinner Option* _____
Snack: *Just Stop Snack Option* _____ *(only when absolutely necessary, see Snack Options page)*
Splurge: *Just Stop Splurge Option* _____ (only if you have less than 20 pounds to lose, see Splurge Options page)

MONDAY

Breakfast: *Just Stop Breakfast Option* _____
Lunch: *Just Stop Lunch Option* _____
Dinner: *Just Stop Dinner Option* _____
Snack: *Just Stop Snack Option* _____ *(only when absolutely necessary, see Snack Options page)*
Splurge: *Just Stop Splurge Option* _____ (only if you have less than 20 pounds to lose, see Splurge Options page)

TUESDAY

Breakfast: *Just Stop Breakfast Option* _____
Lunch: *Just Stop Lunch Option* _____
Dinner: *Just Stop Dinner Option* _____
Snack: *Just Stop Snack Option* _____ *(only when absolutely necessary, see Snack Options page)*
Splurge: *Just Stop Splurge Option* _____ (only if you have less than 20 pounds to lose, see Splurge Options page)

WEDNESDAY

Breakfast: *Just Stop Breakfast Option* _____
Lunch: *Just Stop Lunch Option* _____
Dinner: *Just Stop Dinner Option* _____
Snack: *Just Stop Snack Option* _____ *(only when absolutely necessary, see Snack Options page)*
Splurge: *Just Stop Splurge Option* _____ (only if you have less than 20 pounds to lose, see Splurge Options page)

THURSDAY

Breakfast: *Just Stop Breakfast Option* _____
Lunch: *Just Stop Lunch Option* _____
Dinner: *Just Stop Dinner Option* _____
Snack: *Just Stop Snack Option* _____ *(only when absolutely necessary, see Snack Options page)*
Splurge: *Just Stop Splurge Option* _____ (only if you have less than 20 pounds to lose, see Splurge Options page)

FRIDAY

Breakfast: *Just Stop Breakfast Option* _____
Lunch: *Just Stop Lunch Option* _____
Dinner: *Just Stop Dinner Option* _____
Snack: *Just Stop Snack Option* _____ *(only when absolutely necessary, see Snack Options page)*
Splurge: *Just Stop Splurge Option* _____ (only if you have less than 20 pounds to lose, see Splurge Options page)

(Make copies of this page so you can use it weekly)

Notes

When You're Tempted to Cheat...

Don't do it! Don't reach for the junk food or for *any* kind of food that's not outlined in the Just Stop Eating So Much! Program. You *do* have what it takes to succeed on this. During the more difficult moments, try one of these remedies. They really work!

Your Point of View

You're the one who's going to determine if Just Stop Eating So Much! will be a success for you or not. Don't focus on the foods you're giving up. Instead, look at this as a new beginning to your life – and remember that it's something you're *choosing* to do. Look at the amazing, positive side of what you're doing. You're not giving anything up. You're *choosing* to eat healthier foods in smaller portions and transform your life and your body as a result. This will lead to wonderful things.

So it's not about lack. It's about success and choice. Remember: It's how *you* choose to view the situation. Do you complain, "Oh, I started a new diet and it's hard?" Or do you say "I made a decision to transform my life and I'm really excited about it and know the changes are going to start showing up shortly?" It's your choice. And it's all about attitude. So get yours into gear. And remember: I believe in you! You *can* do this! Tell that to yourself over and over again – because it's true!

Stress-Relieving Breathing Exercise

A lot of times wanting to eat is more about stress, boredom or habit than it is about true hunger. This breathing exercise takes only 5 minutes of your time, but is a really great way to "Change the channel," mentally – whether you're in a panic, stressed out or want to cheat.

1. Put your hand near your nose. Close your right nostril and breathe in through you left nostril.

2. Close your left nostril and breathe out through your right nostril – then breathe in again through your right nostril.

3. Close your right nostril and breathe out through your left nostril – then breathe in again through your left nostril.

4. Repeat this for 5 minutes with your eyes closed (in and out through one nostril, then in and out through the other nostril).

This is very calming and *will* help if you take the time to do it!

When You're Tempted to Cheat... (continued)

Change the "Mental Channel"

As soon as your mind turns to food or thoughts of cheating or breaking down and stopping your Just Stop Eating So Much! efforts, change your mental channel. Don't over analyze, don't over-think. Instead, turn on the TV, reach for a book, start a conversation with a friend (about anything other than food or eating) – do *anything you can* to avoid thinking about cheating or stopping your efforts.

By mentally short-circuiting these thoughts, you take away their power. Over analyzing or talking about them only gives these thoughts more power. That's not what you want to do. Think other thoughts – and think them quickly. It will *really* help.

The Boob Tube

I don't care what anyone says. TV can be fun and can transport you to another place – away from your stressful thoughts about food or your temptations to eat. I'm not suggesting you skip exercise and socializing with actual human beings. But there are times when you'll need to "escape" in order not to cheat (or be tempted to). I suggest joining one of the online DVD rental options and signing up to receive multiple discs of a TV show you've never seen. There's nothing quite as engrossing as watching a drama like *The Sopranos* or a comedy like *The King of Queens* from the beginning. Choose a show you haven't seen, but one that has multiple seasons. Maybe it will be the 13 seasons of *Dallas*. 10 seasons of *Friends*. 6 seasons of *Sex and the City*. Or maybe something more arty that originally aired on public television. The choice is *yours*.

Choose a genre you like and choose a show you haven't seen (or haven't seen much of). One of the great things about online rental services is that they can send you the discs in episode order. Therefore you can rent them without having to purchase the box sets. (Of course, you can also ask for the boxed sets as gifts from friends for your birthday or holidays, too!) It really helps to "lose yourself" in another world of a long running TV series, old or new. Try it!

Here are some resources you can check out for online video rental services:

http://rent-dvds.6starreviews.com

http://www.netflix-dvd.com/

https://www.blockbuster.com

http://www.qwikfliks.com/

When You're Tempted to Cheat… (continued)

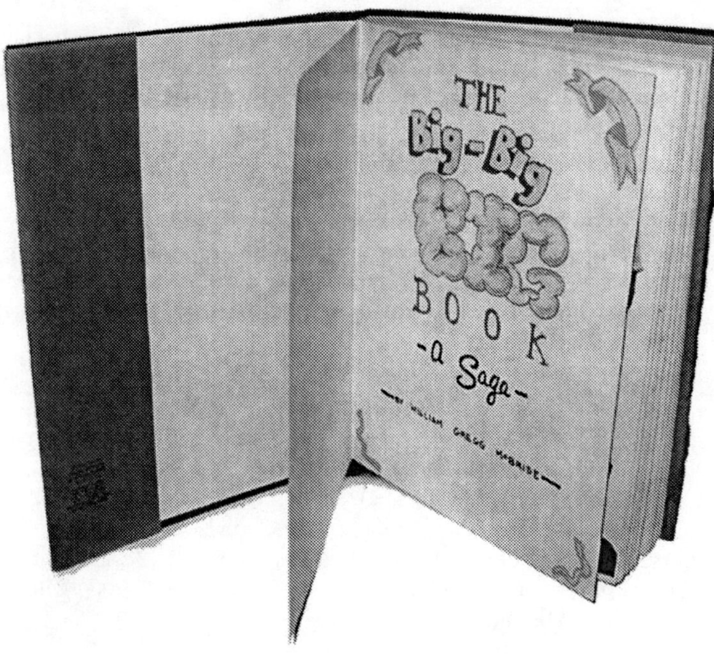

<u>Start Your Own "Just Stop!" Book</u>

As soon as I began my self-made Just Stop! Plan, I bought a large, blank book (meaning blank pages inside). These are easily found in bookstores and art supply stores. I then used this book as a "Success Scrapbook." I would cut out words I found inspiring, articles about health and fitness, pictures from catalogs featuring "thin people clothes" that I wanted to wear, etc. I even put my "Before" picture and my weekly weight into this book.

My book became a real source of inspiration for me and something that I enjoy sharing with people now. After all, I was on a journey. And chronicling that journey was not only therapeutic, but also very inspirational. I suggest you do the same.

Get a book right away. Then keep your eye out for anything you find inspiring (from magazines, catalogs, letters from friends, internet print outs, etc.). There are no rules. This is *your* book. *Your* inspiration! And when you reach your goal, you'll have a testament to your journey and your success. I'd even love to see pictures of your book, so feel free to share them. You can write me at:

gregg@juststopeatingsomuch.com

Just Stop! Stress Busters

Be the center of your own universe

Make a list detailing the people, places and things that throw you off balance. Realize that these things are *all* less important that your well being. You have to take care of yourself before you can take care of anyone else.

Get in touch with what stress really is

Remind yourself that most stressful situations are short-term. They will pass. Certainly some are long-term, of course. When stress presents itself, decide which it is: short-term vs. long-term. That can help you deal with it. And often the first part of *really* handling it is *accepting* it. Stress is a fact of life. It will present itself from time to time.

Don't use food as a crutch

Eating food that's not on the Just Stop! Plan will only lead to more stress. It's a temporary fix that isn't a *fix* at all. Instead, find other, more productive ways to handle your stress – like taking a brisk walk, doing a breathing exercise or watching a favorite movie that will whisk you away, mentally. Sometimes to talk about the stress is really more like encouraging it. Instead, change the channel in your mind – but never do it with food.

Exercise can be key

It's a scientific fact: exercise releases pent-up feelings of annoyance or frustration and actually helps you relax and put things back in perspective. Next time some thing or some*one* ticks you off, instead of losing your temper, lose some more of your belly with some mood-improving working out.

Yoga and meditation offer assistance

A lot of stress can be self-imposed. Therefore, relaxation techniques can help improve your state of mind in a short period of time. Try doing breathing exercises, meditating or taking a long, relaxing yoga class.

Sometimes it's better to step away

Often, confronting the stress isn't worth the effort. For example, a grumpy boss isn't necessarily going to change – and talking to him or her about the issue just might make them even grumpier. Learn to be more like a duck and let the water (stress) roll right off your back. After all, you're on the Just Stop! Plan. And *you're* in charge of your life. Not the grumpy boss.

Reaching Your Goal Weight

Believe it or not, the time will come when you reach your goal weight. You're going to be looking and feeling sensational – and you better promise to send me some before and after pictures so I can celebrate with you!

And surprise! Your Just Stop! Eating Plan will remain in place – even after you've reached your goal. The reason is, if you're like most people on a diet, you've dieted and lost weight before – and then gained it back. It's very important to let your metabolism (and your *body*) know you're serious this time – that you don't want any of the excess weight (that's *blubber*, people!) back.

The Just Stop Eating So Much! Maintenance Plan is simple to follow. You're still going to follow the Eating Plan, picking and choosing Breakfasts, Lunches and Dinners for the appropriate times of day. But you're also going to visit the Splurge Options page, and add 1 Splurge Option per week.

At the end of the first week of maintenance, weigh yourself. If you have remained the same weight, you can now add *two* Splurge Options during the next week. At the end of the second week, if you stay the same weight, you can add *three* Splurge Options. Then, finally, at the end of the fourth week, if you've remained at your goal weight, you can now have *four* Splurge Options a week.

But be careful! You can only have one each of the different Splurge Options outlined. In other words, you can't eat a 'whatever you want meal' (Splurge Option #3) at your favorite restaurant 4 nights a week. That's a once-a-week thing, as are the other Splurge Options.

You will continue to weigh yourself. Any time you rise above your goal weight, even just a pound or two, *cut out all Splurge Options* and stick to the basic Just Stop Eating So Much! Plan until you're back down at your goal.

Remember, you'll have worked hard to achieve this incredible goal. Now, we want to make sure you stay at that goal.

Also, remember to keep up and add to and change out your exercise options, as well! Feeling good and being healthy on the inside is as important and looking good on the outside.

When You've Reached Your Goal

I want to hear from you! Email me and tell me about your success!

gregg@juststopeatingsomuch.com

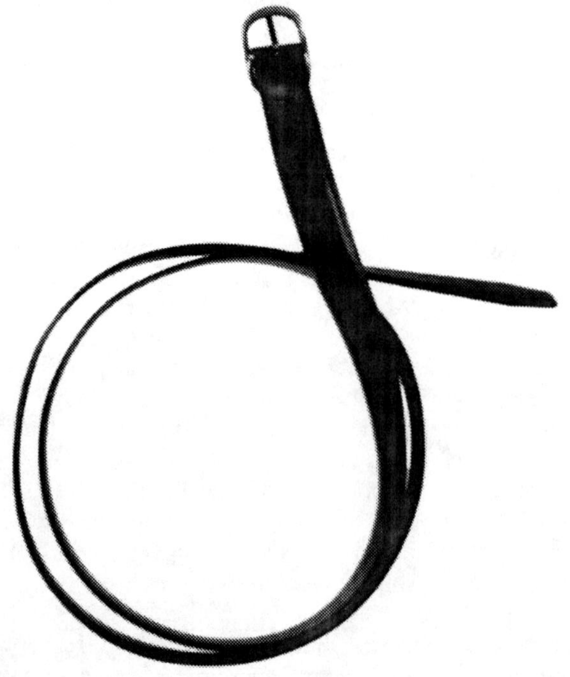

Tough Love

You're more powerful than food!

I know ice cream can be tempting. I know cookies can tease. I know that food can be very addictive. And that exercise can be a time-consuming drag. But so what? It's time for a little tough love. And that's where the whole conceit behind Just Stop Eating So Much! kicks in!

You've made excuses in your past as to why you had to "cheat" on your diet or not exercise or just have that "one cookie." And look at you. You're not happy with how you look, you're feeling frustrated about how your clothes fit, you could even be facing ill health – not to mention tough relationships and other obstacles that overweight people must face in our society.

But those days are over! You *can* do this. The change starts now – this very day. Don't put it off any longer! If you take the crybaby approach and feel sorry for yourself, you're going to fail. But I think I know you better than that. I know you can do this. I know you have what it takes. This is the day the coddling stops. No more feeling sorry for yourself. No more longing for the foods that have contributed to your poor appearance and poor health.

Just answer this: ***Do you want to be thin or fat?*** (It's that simple!)

Kick your blubber to the curb. I took off more than 250 pounds in less than a year following this program. And I've kept the weight off for over 10 years. Without surgery. Without pills. Without fads. Without personal trainers. Without special foods. Without expensive meal delivery services.

The time is now. And it's time to **Just Stop Eating So Much!** Tough love? Maybe? But the *real* truth? *Definitely*!

A Final Thought:

There's something I can guarantee you. It's something I've promised others that I've helped succeed on the Just Stop Eating So Much! Plan. Sure, they might not have believed me at first. But no matter what, in the end, when they reach their goals, they always repeat these words back to me and tell me I was right. I'm going to share these words with you, too – because they're *true*!

Nothing tastes as good as being thin feels!

Believe it! Live it! *Do it*!

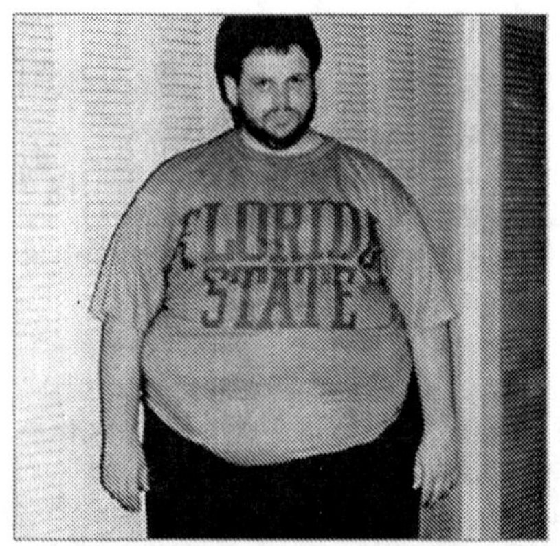
FLORIDA
STATE

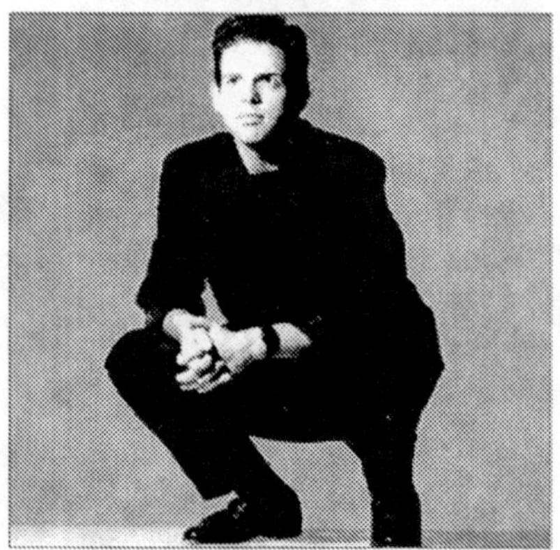

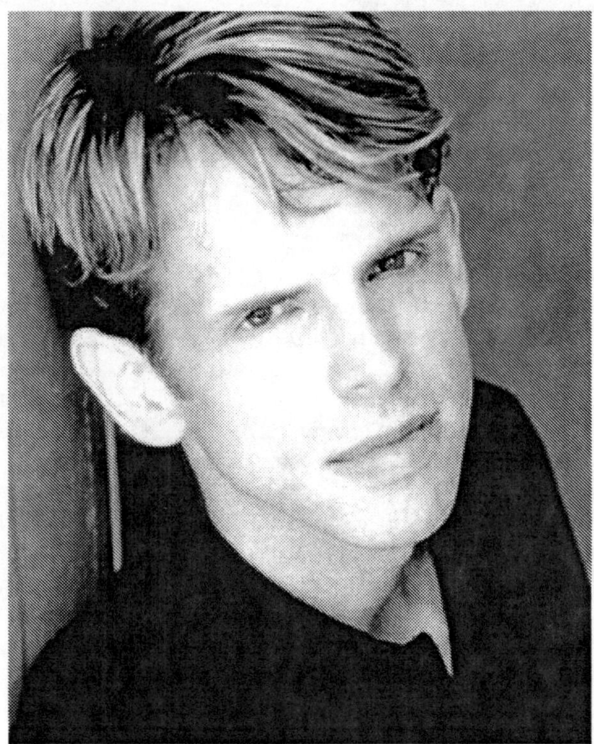

Meet the creator of Just Stop Eating So Much!, Gregg McBride

A former advertising Creative Director, Gregg McBride is now a writer residing in Los Angeles, California. Gregg's screenwriting credits include "Happily Never After" (Disney), "Have a Nice Life" (MTV Films), "Epicenter" (Sci-Fi Channel), "Before & After" (USA), "Stepmonster" (an original TV series he created for MTV) and more.

More relevant to this project, Gregg has been fighting the battle of the bulge for his entire life. As early as the first grade, he was called "fat" and put on strict diets by his parents, doctors and other professionals. Everyone wondered what was wrong with him when all of the diets failed. Gregg continued to try and lose weight as an adult, joining weight loss groups, paying hundreds – even thousands – of dollars to organizations and programs that promised quick fixes to his lifelong problem.

Upon graduating from college, Gregg tipped the scales at 450 pounds and would literally be left breathless from having a conversation on the phone.

It's when Gregg stopped looking for a quick fix and started using common sense that he had a breakthrough – one that his friends, colleagues and countless strangers have begged him to share once they learned that this now thin, healthy and attractive young man used to weigh as much as he did and used to be so large that he literally broke a movie theater seat (while on a date, no less).

Just Stop Eating So Much! is a work of passion for Gregg – a work that he really cares about and really wants to share. Because he *really knows* what it's like to be trapped in a body with a massive layer of blubber surrounding it – trapped in the "big and tall" store, searching for pants with a size 60-inch waist when shopping for clothes – and trapped into thinking that spending thousands upon thousands of dollars or even having his body altered through surgery was the only way to a normal, happy, healthy life.

Gregg has spent his entire life exploring his passion as a writer. First with crayons (usually on walls), then in "novels" he wrote during school (he usually never got past chapter 3), later in advertising and now for the screen.

Gregg was also a featured contributor to the highly successful non-fiction book, *Ask the Pros: Screenwriting – 101 Questions Answered by Industry Professionals.*

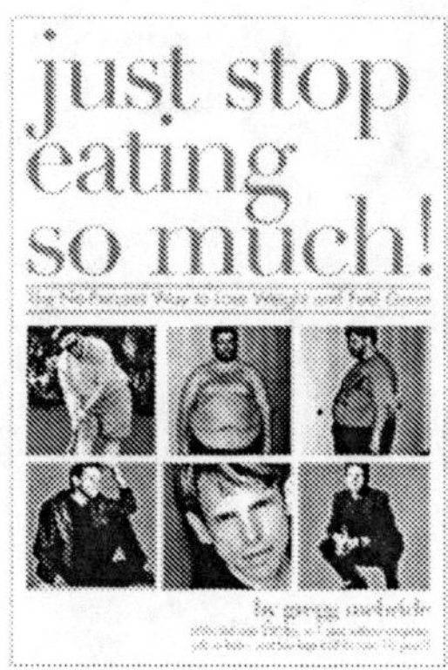

Do you want to be part of the Just Stop Eating So Much! Phenomenon?

Visit Just Stop! Online

Visit the Just Stop Eating So Much! website to get additional tips, strategies, recipes and more. You can also chat and interact with other Just Stop! Plan Members and even interact with Gregg, himself. We look forward to interacting with you online:

http://juststopeatingsomuch.com/

Help Others, Help Yourself

Send your questions, comments and ideas to Gregg at the email address below. By doing so, you just might be featured on the Just Stop Eating So Much! website, in one of our eNewsletters or even in a future Just Stop Eating So Much! Book.

Along with whatever you want to ask (or share), be sure to include a little biographical information about yourself (even a picture, if you'd like). Don't worry, we'll only refer to you by first name and location (unless you specifically request to remain anonymous). Gregg looks forward to hearing from you.

You can email Gregg at: gregg@juststopeatingsomuch.com

(Please note that sending anything to the email address above signifies your agreement to your comments, questions or ideas being used in future Just Stop Eating So Much! material. If you include a picture or pictures in your email, you agree we can use it/them in print and online, as well. Thank you.)

Printed in the United States
102998LV00004B/250-297/A